The 3 Pillars of Strength:

Improving Your Physical, Mental and Spiritual Fitness

By Jeffrey White

Published by Richter Publishing LLC www.richterpublishing.com

Editors: Casey Cavanagh & Ke'Shawnda Chambers

Copyright © 2015 Jeffrey White

ISBN:0692424776
ISBN-13:9780692424773

DISCLAIMER

This book is designed to provide information on health and fitness only. This information is provided and sold with the knowledge that the publisher and author do not offer any legal or medical advice. In the case of a need for any such expertise, consult with the appropriate professional. This book does not contain all information available on the subject. This book has not been created to be specific to any individual's or organization's situation or needs. Every effort has been made to make this book as accurate as possible. However, there may be typographical and/ or content errors. Therefore, this book should serve only as a general guide and not as the ultimate source of subject information. This book contains information that might be dated and is intended only to educate and entertain. The author and publisher shall have no liability or responsibility to any person or entity regarding any loss or damage incurred, or alleged to have incurred, directly or indirectly, by the information contained in this book. You hereby agree to be bound by this disclaimer or you may return this book within the guarantee time period for a full refund. In the interest of full disclosure, this book contains affiliate links that might pay the author or publisher a commission upon any purchase from the company. While the author and publisher take no responsibility for the business practices of these companies and or the performance of any product or service, the author or publisher has used the product or service and makes a recommendation in good faith based on that experience. All characters appearing in this work are fictitious. Any resemblance to real persons, living or dead, is purely coincidental.

Table of Contents

ACKNOWLEDGMENTS

First and foremost, I'd like to thank God for giving me the strength to write this book and for blessing my life thus far. Without His grace and mercy I wouldn't be here.

I'd also like to thank Tara Richter and her staff at Richter Publishing for doing an outstanding job in helping me bring this project to life.

I want to acknowledge several people who influenced me to write this book. I have known the majority of them my entire life, and I appreciate everything they have taught me over the years. Their support has been tremendous and I appreciate each of them.

My father was not in my life, but I was fortunate enough to have 3 strong male role models when I needed them the most. They treated me like a son when they really didn't have to and I appreciate that. So to my uncles George Edwards, Nathanial Edwards (in memoriam) and Phillip Edwards, I thank you. Not only did you give me kind words of encouragement over the years, you led by example. You showed me how to be a responsible adult with your actions. I can't thank you enough.

Even though I'm an only child, I don't feel that way as I have cousins who I considered my brothers and sisters growing up. I looked up to them and they ALWAYS looked out for me. Thank you Brian Ross and Jerry Foster for being the big brothers I never had. To my cousins Elliott, Timothy, Rochelle and Adrienna Edwards, many of my childhood memories include you all. I never considered us cousins. I always thought of you as my little brothers and sisters!

I have been very fortunate and thankful to have some very strong women role models in my life. Charlotte Shaw, Nathalie Moore (both (in memoriam) and Pam Harrison are three women I have a tremendous amount of respect for and love dearly. As I said before, I'm an only child, but Kendra Williams is TRULY my sister. She would take care of me when we were younger and she can **still** put me in my place. I LOVE YOU KENDRA!

I have a pretty large extended family and unfortunately I can't name them all. So to the rest of my family: The Noel's, Foster's, Williams, Steptore's, Harrisons, and Edwards, I thank you for helping me have a happy, memorable, and fun childhood! I have a great family and I'm PROUD to say I'm related to each and every one of you!

As great as my childhood was, college was the best time of my life. College laid the foundation for many of the healthy habits I have today, and I also became a member of my new family, The Federation!

I only wish people had friends like these. We've been there for each other in good times and bad for over 20 years. Going to Illinois State University was one of the best decisions I ever made because it allowed me to meet *The FEDERATION:* Clifton "A-Train" Boyd, Don "Lord" Reed, Norman "Dawg Team" Ross, Michael "Cymone" Turner, Michael "Ice Mike" McCreary, Lovise "5Linx" Jiles, Darren "Double D" Davis, Reggie "Doc Wild" Hopkins, Leonard Alonzo Cain, and my dearly departed brothers Carlos Phelix, Jarrett Moore, and Trent Leggs. These are truly my brothers!

Moving to Tampa was one of the best decisions I ever made, as it was here I met my wife. To my wife Monica and son Little Jeffrey, without you two I'm nothing. Family is everything, and I'm honored to be blessed with you both. Nothing comes above family and we are taking this journey together, as a family. I want to make you both proud! The best is yet to come for us!

I have been fortunate enough to become part of a family here in Tampa that is very close knit and supportive. If you need something, they are there for you without hesitation. My father in law, Deacon Alphonso Adams is a man who I have the utmost respect for. To my "new" family: Deaconess Jaqueline Adams, Mark, Sonia, Gino, Lois, Cynthia, and Kay, thank you for bringing me into the fold!

Last but certainly not least is my mother, Patricia White Sterling. I can't stress how much love and respect I have for her, a single mother raising a black male on the south side of Chicago. To this day, I'm amazed at her strength and so thankful she kept me focused on school and not getting in trouble. She was a beautiful person inside and out, and I'm proud to be her son. Her love and guidance is why I was able to write this book, and for that I am truly thankful.

DEDICATION

Sometimes you have to go for it. The path you're currently on is headed nowhere, and the path you WANT to take is so foggy you can't see 30 feet in front of you. You THINK a path is there, but you don't know for sure. Should you go for it, or just stay on your current path?

You're at the point where you throw caution to the wind and simply say, "I'm going for it. I'm taking this path of uncertainty and I will let it take me wherever it leads me. I'm not afraid and will accept the challenges as they come towards me."

This book is my new path and writing it is the foggiest stretch of road I've ever been on. I have no idea where it will take me, but that's where I'm going, and I'm not looking back. That old path was leading me to a lifetime of regret and unfulfilled hopes and dreams. I'm headed in a new direction. I refuse to let someone else control my happiness and destiny. Not anymore.

I'd like to thank my wife Monica for her support in writing this book, as well as encouraging me to go after my dreams.

I'd also like to thank the great friends who inspired me to write this book by sharing their stories with me over the years. I was listening and maybe, just maybe, this book will inspire you to embark on a new path as well. If I can, you can too!

To my son Little Jeffrey, you're too young to read these words right now, but one day you'll be old enough to understand. Just know that I love you, and I simply want to make you proud. You can do whatever you set your mind to. I have your back and will ALWAYS be here for you! It's time, LJ. It's TIME!

INTRODUCTION: IT'S TIME

It's time to be the best person you can be. It's time for YOU to reach your FULL potential.

It's time to tap into ALL your unique traits and talents that can propel you to greatness.

It's time to face all the challenges and obstacles this world will throw at you with the quiet confidence that you CAN and WILL overcome.

It's time to understand that, at your disposal, you have the tools needed to be the best you can be.

It's time to realize that the ONLY thing really holding you back from achieving your dreams is YOU.

It's time to realize that you are a very complex and intricate individual, and to perform at your best, you must work on ALL aspects of your life.

It's time to believe *WITHOUT A DOUBT* that no matter who you are or what stage of life you're in, you still have the ability to reach heights you never thought possible.

We've all heard this before, but you may wonder, "What does it all mean?"

Many of us are living our life like it is a giant jigsaw puzzle; some pieces are in place, while others are lost or still jumbled. To be the best you can be, all your pieces must be in place, and it's up to you to put them in the appropriate sections.

For example: Being a successful, wealthy person isn't very enjoyable if you are ill or have health problems such as diabetes, high blood pressure, or a heart condition.

No matter how talented or gifted a person is, they will never reach their full potential if they have low self-esteem, doubt their own abilities, or are easily discouraged by others.

If a person is full of anger and resentment, they will have a difficult time enjoying life and living it to the fullest, as they may be preoccupied with all the wrongs done to them.

While these are separate examples, it's important to understand that shortcomings in one aspect of your life could have a ripple effect and drastically affect other aspects.

The purpose of this book is to help you become physically, mentally and spiritually fit— simultaneously—with each aspect of fitness having its own section.

Many of us tend to focus on our spirituality, while neglecting our physical health.

Others demean themselves and lose all self-respect in the quest for money or success.

Instead of dealing with their issues head on, some will abuse alcohol, drugs, or engage in other harmful activities in hopes of avoiding the situation.

This is just a few of the ways we may be out of balance, and it's up to you to put all the pieces together!

You only have one life, and it's up to YOU to live it to the fullest. No one else can do it for you, so that means it's TIME to make things right!

PILLAR I

PHYSICAL FITNESS

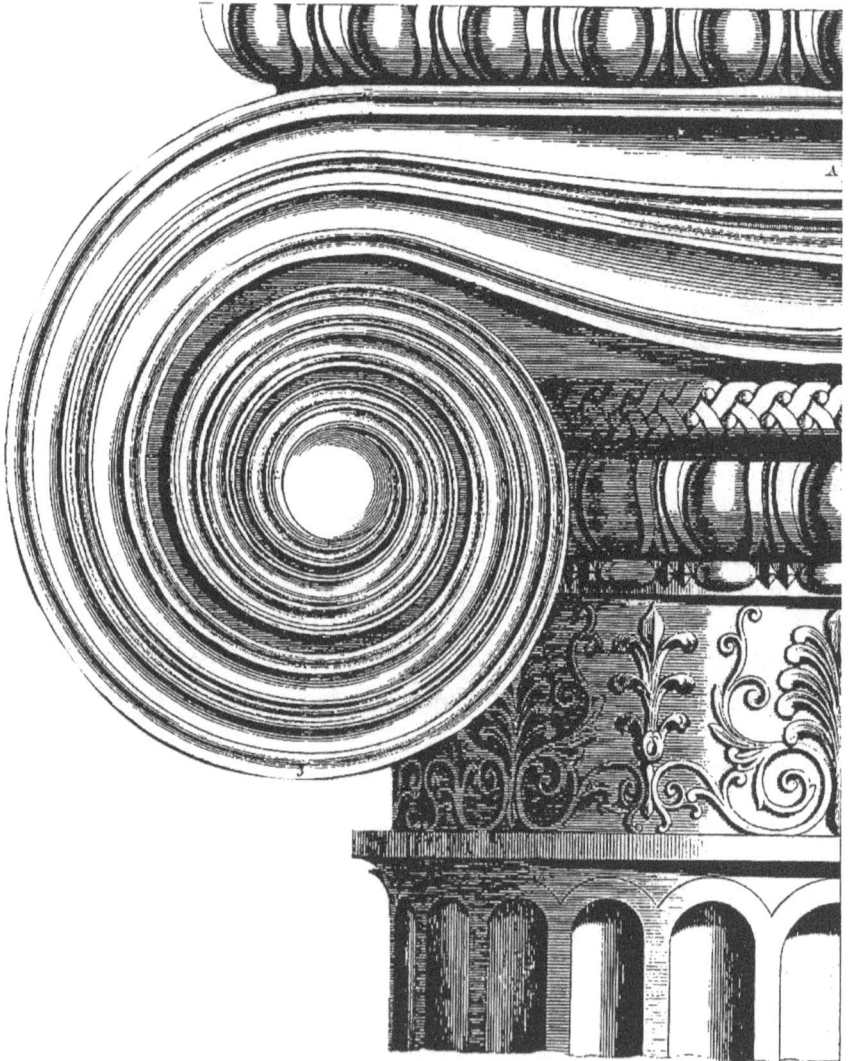

This section highlights the importance of being physically fit and finding exercises that work best for YOU, not just what's popular right now. The exercises your best friends are doing may or may not yield the same results for you, and it's important to understand this.

In this section there's also a mention of mental fitness, because in order to be your best physically, you must be mentally strong.

When reading this section, it's all about YOU. Don't worry about what others are doing or compare yourself to them. We all progress at our own pace, so focus on your own self-improvement.

CHAPTER 1: FITNESS TRENDS

Many people ask me what the "best" exercise program is, or what I think of XYZ training system. They are eager to try something new that will give them FAST results.

As a society, we are always looking for the "next best thing," or the quick fix. Many manufacturers use buzz words like "cutting edge" or "new and improved" to get people's attention and make you THINK this new "revolutionary product" is the wave of the future and is that much better than everything else that's out there.

These companies will get a spokesperson who is currently popular to pitch their product and/or spend a tremendous amount of money on advertising to get the word out about it.

Since people are always looking for something new, they are eager to try it. But can the product really do what they claim? Is it really better than what's currently out?

People are always looking for the next big thing, be it in fashion or fitness:

Jazzercise (1969)
Tae Bo (1976)
Step Aerobics (1989)
Thighmaster (1990)

The Bodyblade (1991)
The Hawaii Chair (2007)
Shake Weight (2010)
Ab Rocket (exact date unknown)

Jack LaLanne Exercise Plan (1936)
Joe Weider Weider Nutrition (1936)
Richard Simmons Sweatin to the Oldies (1980)
Jane Fonda The Jane Fonda Workout Plan (1982))
Shaun T Insanity (2009)

Then there are the diet trends. The following list is a sample of popular diets over the years:

Vinegar and Water Diet
Made popular in 1820 by Lord Byron. In order to cleanse his body he would drink vinegar and water daily (in addition to a cup of tea with a raw egg mixed in). Side effects included vomiting and diarrhea.

 Harvey-Banting Low Carb Diet Created in 1863. Diet described in the booklet Letter on Corpulence that recommended four meals per day, consisting of meat, greens, fruits, and dry wine. The emphasis was on avoiding sugar, saccharine matter, starch, beer, milk and butter.

Cigarette Diet
An advertising campaign began this diet in the 1920s. Created by Albert Lasker for Lucky Strike cigarettes, "Reach for a Lucky" was aimed especially at women, and cited nicotine's alleged weight-loss properties to make it more acceptable for women to smoke their product.

The Inuit Diet Created in 1928. All the caribou, raw fish and whale blubber you can eat.

Bananas and Skim Milk Diet
In 1934, this diet was advertised so that the United Fruit Company could sell more bananas. Dr. George Harrop looked at fat-free skim milk and potassium-rich bananas and created a new weight-loss plan.

Drinking Man's Diet
Created in 1964 by Robert Cameron. The plan was heavy on steaks, rich cheeses and other fatty foods, with the kicker being that you can drink as much hard liquor as you like, because it contains only trace amounts of carbohydrates. The director of Harvard's School of Nutrition decried the diet in an article, calling it "mass murder."

Paleolithic Diet Created in the 1970's by gastroenterologist Walter Voegtlin, but was made popular in 2002 by Loren Cordain. This diet is based on the food humans' ancient ancestors might likely have eaten, such as meat, nuts and berries. It is also known also known as the paleo diet or caveman diet.

Lean Cuisine was created as a healthier alternative to Stouffer's frozen meals. Because of the word "lean," the FDA requires the product to meet the "lean" criteria of less than 10 grams of fat, 4.5 grams or less of saturated fat, and less than 95 milligrams of cholesterol.

Beverly Hills Diet
In her book, named after the diet, Judy Mazel advocated a slx-week-long program, beginning with 10 days of specific fruits in a certain order.

Dukan Diet
Founded by Frenchman Pierre Dukan, the diet was in existence for 30 years before the book was published and became an instant bestseller. It is similar to the Atkins diet, but does not allow fats and oils, and insists on the daily consumption of oat bran.

Coconut Diet
This diet begins with a 21-day kickoff where one must avoid fruit, alcohol, dairy, sugar and caffeine. Three meals a day of vegetables, nuts and lean proteins must include 2 tablespoons of extra virgin coconut oil, which speeds up your metabolism.

South Beach Diet Created in 1995 by cardiologist Dr. Arthur Agatston. The diet emphasized eating high-fiber, low-glycemic carbohydrates, unsaturated fats, and lean protein, and categorizes carbohydrates and fats as "good" or "bad."

Dexatrim Developed in the 1970's by Thompson Medical

Nutrisystem Created in 1972 by Harold Katz

Scarsdale Diet Created in the 1970's by Dr. Herman Tarnower

Lipozene Created in 2006 by the Obesity Research Institute LLC

So when people ask me about the "best" exercises, instead of giving people a direct answer, I ask them a few simple, rhetorical questions:

What was the fitness rage last year? 5 years ago? 10 years ago? What was the style of dress? Hairstyle?

Fashion Trends:

Saggy pants
Jerry Curls
Bell bottoms
Cross Colours
White tees
FUBU
Bart Simpson Tees
Skinny jeans
Leather pants
Crocs
Big Hair
Grunge look
Multi-colored tube socks
Tight basketball shorts, etc.

The point here is that trends come and go. Some of the items on this list you might be aware of, some you may not. (Some may be collecting dust in your basement as you read this!) What's hot today can be gone tomorrow. It doesn't matter if it's the latest fashion, exercise, or diet trend.

People must remember: THE NUMBER ONE GOAL OF A COMPANY IS TO MAKE MONEY, and they will do whatever it takes to make a profit.

Some companies really are trying to deliver a product that is designed to help you as advertised, but others, unfortunately, are not. They are simply trying to generate a profit, as they feel this is what the buying public wants to spend their money on. When the public is ready for a new product, those companies will gladly deliver it.

Again, it doesn't matter if it's the latest fashion, exercise, or diet trend.

Looking at the list of health products above, decide for yourself which of these were genuinely good products, and which were fads. At the time, these products weren't considered "fads." They were considered "revolutionary."
As you look at the list, ask yourself: *What products out TODAY will be here 5 years from now? 10 years from now?*

Which of these diets and meal plans are designed to help me become a healthier person, and which are designed to help the creator retire early?

There's nothing wrong with seeking new and exciting products that will improve your quality of life, but sometimes we tend to neglect the tried and true methods that have been around for hundreds of years.

Many look at fitness in the same light as technology, but can't fully compare the two. It's safe to assume the latest smartphone or television is much more advanced than the model that's 5 years old.

The improvements in communication, such as in our mobile phones and the internet, have made our lives that much easier. Thirty years ago, speaking to someone on the other side of the world would be very expensive via phone, or very slow via letter.

When it comes to technology, many of us can't wait to "upgrade"— whether it be our phone, television, or even our vehicle.

However, when it comes to fitness, this doesn't always apply. At least, it shouldn't. For example, the basic exercises people used to stay fit, such as jogging, push-ups and cycling, still have the same health benefits now as they did decades ago. Our bodies are still pretty much the same. As a society, we are heavier than previous generations, but we still respond to those exercises the same way our grandparents did.

Some things stand the test of time, while others come and go, never to return.

Many believe the new diet plan or fitness machine is the answer, and are willing to spend huge sums of money on it, but it's all for naught.

According to the U. S. Food and Drug Administration (FDA), in 1992 Americans spent an estimated $30 billion on all types of diet programs and products, including diet foods and drinks.

Marketdata, a market research firm that has tracked diet products and programs since 1989, release its findings in a biennial study, "The U.S. Weight Loss & Diet Control Market." In a its 2007 study, they estimated the size of the U.S. weight loss market at $55 billion. It is now estimated to have reached over $60 billion.

You'd think that, with all that money being spent, we'd be losing weight and getting in better shape, but that's not the case.

Among 2007 Behavioral Risk Factor Surveillance System (BRFSS) respondents it was found that the average American adult is more than 24 pounds heavier today than in 1960.

Even though we are spending BILLIONS OF DOLLARS on fitness and weight loss products, obesity rates are steadily increasing. More than two-thirds (68.7%) of American adults are either overweight or obese, with African American adults having the highest rates of obesity at 72.7%.

U.S. Overweight and Obesity Rates for Adults by Race/Ethnicity

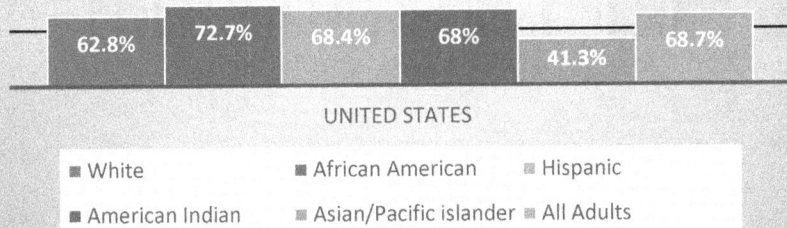

| 62.8% | 72.7% | 68.4% | 68% | 41.3% | 68.7% |

UNITED STATES

- White
- African American
- Hispanic
- American Indian
- Asian/Pacific islander
- All Adults

The obesity prevalence was higher in the South (27.3%) and Midwest (26.5%) and lower in the Northeast (24.4%) and West (23.1%).

U.S. Obesity Rates By Region

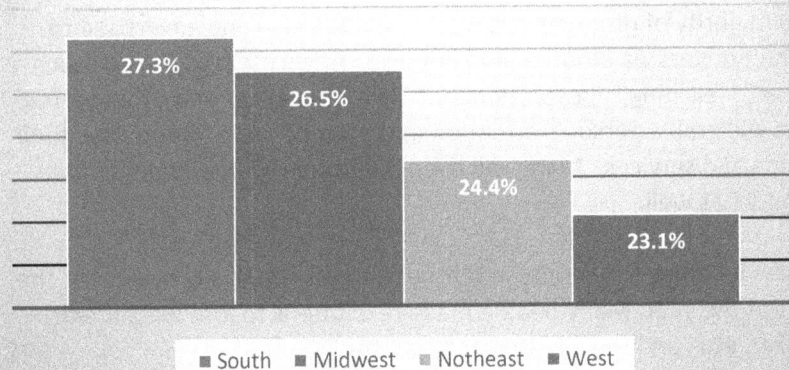

| 27.3% | 26.5% | 24.4% | 23.1% |

- South
- Midwest
- Notheast
- West

It should also be noted that adult obesity rates are rising around the world. According to the World Health Organization, worldwide obesity has more than doubled since 1980. Here's a chart showing the obesity rates in various countries:

Adult Obesity Rates by Country

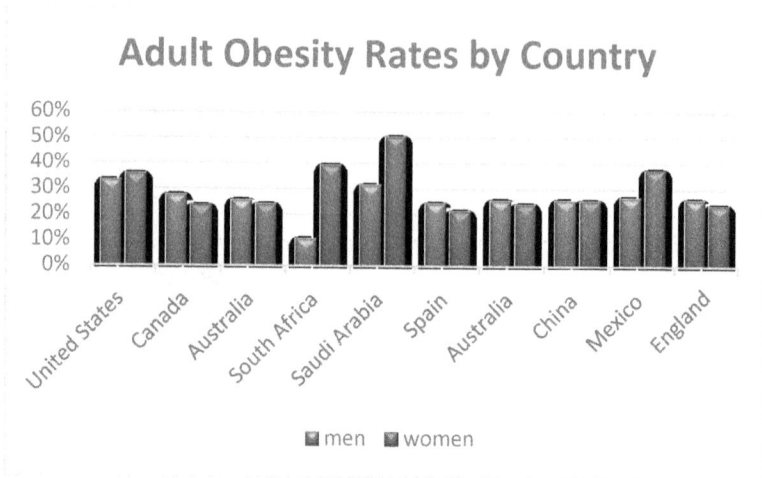

men   women

This is a problem that is not going away anytime soon, and people around the world are looking for products that will assist them with their weight loss goals. However, it's not the new product that will help you become fit, it's your mindset and your desire to work hard to achieve your goals that will help.

The majority of products out there are marketed and advertised to attract buyers via emotion and impulse. Advertisers use words such as "new," "exciting," "revolutionary," "fast," "results," and other words that will grab a person's attention and prompt them to purchase their goods and services. Many will even hire a celebrity to endorse their product as well.

When it comes to exercise and fitness, this is especially evident at the first of the year. Many people make resolutions to lose weight, eat better, etc., and the advertisers know this.

Remember: A business's number one goal is to make money, so companies will invest millions of dollars on advertising to attract consumers. There is a strong push in December and January to tap into the emotional needs of those looking to get fit.

If there was a "Black Friday" for the fitness industry, it would be January

1st. Gym memberships and fitness equipment go on sale. Fitness and weight loss challenges are plentiful. People are ready to make changes in their lives and are spending a lot of money to do it.

Fitness has been a growing industry during the past couple of decades. According to the International Health, Racquet & Sportsclub Association (IHRSA), the revenue of the U.S. health club industry reached $21.4 billion as memberships totaled 51.4 million in 2011.

Unfortunately, people aren't using the gyms as much as they should, as it is estimated that 60% of gym memberships go unused, and New Year's resolutions are just as bad. By mid-January, only 60% of people are still on track. By June, the numbers drop to approximately 40%, and by the end of the year, only 8% of people meet their New Year's resolution goal.

It's a vicious cycle. Let's break it down:

Consumer not happy with weight, physical condition, etc. vows to make changes.
Consumer seeks to find new product that will help them achieve results (fast and with minimal effort).

Companies look to capitalize on this need/want by creating products that will entice consumers to buy.

Consumer becomes excited and purchases new product.
Consumer discovers it will take longer and is harder than expected.
Consumer gets discouraged and gives up.
Products collect dust; gym memberships go unused.
Companies begin to market new products and offer sales on existing products.

This cycle repeats year after year for many people, but it doesn't have to. Many of the resolutions being discussed here are physical, but mental changes must be made as well. Companies are offering products that are designed to help you physically, but the mental aspect is being neglected. Very few physical changes can be made without being mentally prepared to MAKE the changes, as well as the ability to stay focused when it takes longer than expected to lose the weight. That company is selling a PRODUCT, but it's up to YOU to change your MINDSET to make that product work (if it even works)!

Many of these companies WANT you to keep coming back year after year, testing new product after new product, because that's how they make their money. They are counting on you to get discouraged and quit, only to get motivated the next year to try their new "revolutionary product."

But we're not doing that. Not this time. The first step is to have a general understanding of what's really going on, and to implement a plan of action to get the results you desire—a plan of action that will WORK. This means we have to focus on the mental aspect of getting physically fit, which leads us into the next section: Looking Fit vs. Being Fit.

CHAPTER 2: LOOKING FIT VS. BEING FIT: WHAT'S THE DIFFERENCE?

It seems as though many people are more concerned with having a certain look as it pertains to fitness. They want the flat abs and the sexy muscles. They want that perfect body. And who can blame them? Turn on the television or open a magazine and you'll see that practically all the models have "perfect bodies."

Not only do they have the perfect body, but they look healthy and VERY happy! They're standing there in the perfect pose, looking happy and confident, without a care in the world!

Having that "fit" look is something that many are now trying to attain, and they are using many methods to get the look they want. Some are exercising religiously; others are on diets; and some resort to plastic (cosmetic) surgery.

Make no mistake: Attempting to look our best isn't a bad thing. There's nothing wrong with trying to improve yourself. We ALL should strive to be better in some way; that's the basic premise of this book.

Unfortunately, what we want and the METHODS we use may not be the best for us.

Some of the things we're doing to ourselves may be doing more harm than good.

As discussed in the previous section, some are chasing fads and trends that really don't work, or simply aren't good for them.

For some, getting those flat abs and lean, ripped muscles mean long hours in the gym and really watching their calories.

This is good, as we need exercise and sensible eating to be the best we can be.

The problem occurs when they aren't getting the vitamins and minerals their body needs to be in the best shape.

In their quest to look their best on the OUTSIDE, they are sacrificing their health on the INSIDE.

It's great to keep your car shiny and looking good, washing it every Saturday, but if you're not getting the oil changes and tune-ups as required, what good is it?

It's just a matter of time before that clean and shiny car breaks down, leaving you stranded on the side of the road.

It's the same with your body. Just like that car, you can look FANTASTIC on the outside, but inside you could be full of illness and disease that can't be seen so easily.

You could have a headache, high blood pressure, cancer, diabetes, heart conditions, AIDS, etc.

There are countless ailments a person could have that aren't blatantly obvious just by looking at them, especially if they are in the early stages.

The human body is a finely tuned machine that needs a variety of vitamins and nutrients to work at its peak. A person who is determined to lose weight by extreme dieting is bound to be malnourished at some point.

And over the long term, those nutritional deficiencies could damage a person's immune system, thus increasing their risk of becoming ill and having some of the ailments listed above.

These deficiencies could show up in ways people may not expect.

The Center for Disease Control and Prevention (CDC) has written extensively about this and many other health topics. According to a 2012 Second National Report on Biochemical Indicators of Diet and Nutrition by the CDC, *"Overall, the U.S. population has good levels of vitamins A and D and folate in the body, but some groups still need to increase their levels of vitamin D and iron."*

It's also suggested that we eat 5-9 servings of fruits and veggies daily, but according to 2009 statistics, no state or territory in the U.S. has over 50% of their population consuming fruit more than twice a day, or vegetables 3 times a day. It actually has decreased a bit.

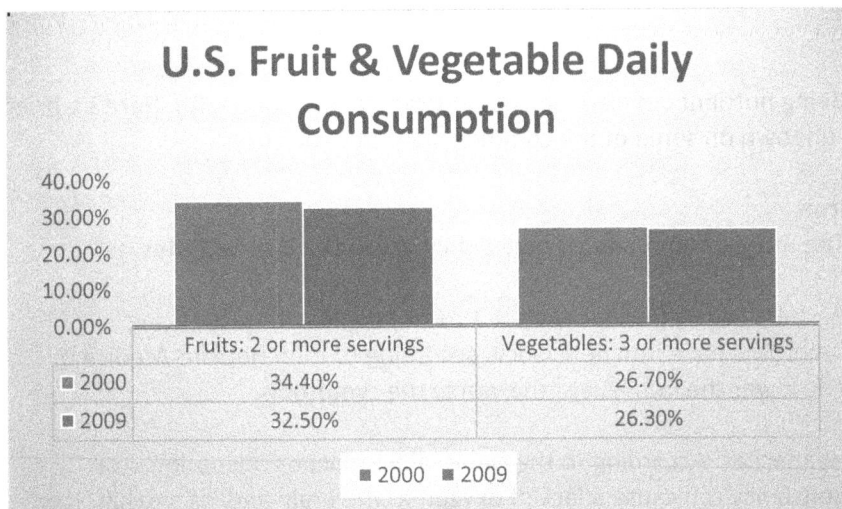

U.S. Fruit & Vegetable Daily Consumption

	Fruits: 2 or more servings	Vegetables: 3 or more servings
2000	34.40%	26.70%
2009	32.50%	26.30%

■ 2000 ■ 2009

The point here is simple: Many of us are already not getting the nutrients we need, and those who are cutting back on calories to achieve a certain look risk becoming even more nutrient deficient.

There are many studies coming up with similar conclusions. According to a 2012 report from Consumer Lab, Americans were in good health overall, but were deficient in a few vitamins and minerals:

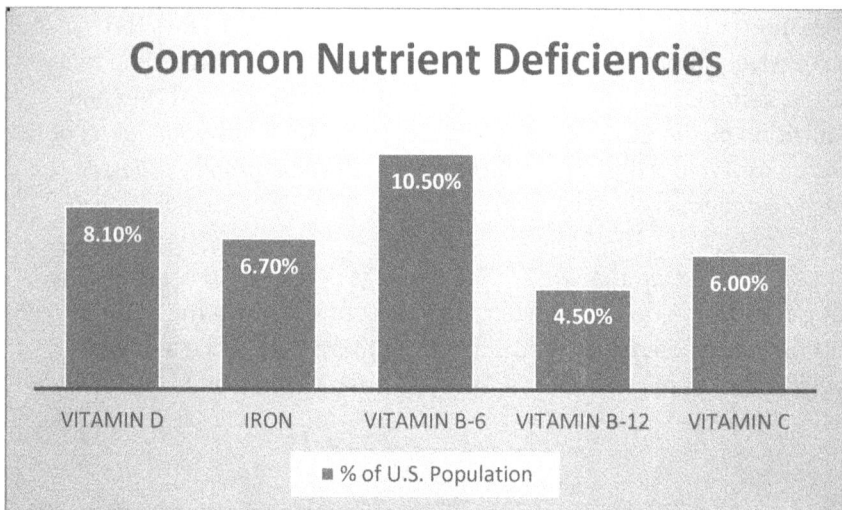

Common Nutrient Deficiencies

Nutrient	% of U.S. Population
VITAMIN D	8.10%
IRON	6.70%
VITAMIN B-6	10.50%
VITAMIN B-12	4.50%
VITAMIN C	6.00%

■ % of U.S. Population

Being nutrient deficient can be detrimental to your health. Here's a brief rundown on some of the common signs of deficiency:

Iron
The most common nutritional deficiency in the United States.

Restless Leg Syndrome. About 15% of people with restless leg syndrome have iron deficiency, according to John Hopkins Medicine. The lower the iron levels, the worse the symptoms.

Headaches. According to the National Headache Foundation, iron deficiency can cause a lack of oxygen to the brain and, as a result, the arteries can swell, causing headaches.

Vitamin A

Signs and symptoms of vitamin deficiency anemia include:
Fatigue
Shortness of breath
Dizziness
Pale or yellowish skin
Irregular heartbeats
Weight loss
Numbness or tingling in hands and feet
Muscle weakness

Vitamin D deficiency

Symptoms of bone pain and muscle weakness could signal a vitamin D deficiency. Low blood levels of the vitamin have been associated with the following:

Increased risk of death from cardiovascular disease
Cognitive impairment in older adults
Severe asthma in children
Cancer

This is just a small sample of the potential vitamin deficiencies and how they affect the body. It's important that a person doesn't sacrifice getting the vital nutrients they need just to have flat abs or be considered the "ideal" shape or size.

It's also very a possible a person could be taking medicine for something that could be remedied by simply getting the recommended nutrients.

Using iron as an example, how many people are experiencing headaches because they have low iron levels? How many of those people are talking medication to deal with those headaches? How many of those people don't know their low iron levels are the cause?

Remember: That "shiny car" does you no good if it's stalled on the side of the road. Don't let your quest to look fit be detrimental to your health. That 6 pack is nice, but it's not more important than passing a physical or getting a clean bill of health.

Next, we'll detail how a person who we THINK is fit really isn't as fit as they appear, and how some are actually FITTER than you thought. Looks really CAN be deceiving...

CHAPTER 3: LOOKS CAN BE DECEIVING

If you ask people what they consider to be a healthy look or physique, they will more than likely pick one particular look or body type over others. On the flip side, they will think certain body types aren't as healthy as others.

It's time to shatter this myth.

As far as "looking" fit, I'll use bodybuilding as an extreme example. We all know bodybuilders are very meticulous with their diets and exercise. They will count every single calorie and change their diets throughout the season.

The week before a big contest is the most critical, as they have to really tweak their diets so all their muscles are clearly visible for the judges to see.

They're already on strict diets, but now, a week before the show, they cut their calories even more. Their water intake decreases to make the striations in their muscles even MORE visible.

On average, male bodybuilders may be around 9-10% body fat year round, but on the day of the competition they are around 4%.

For the women, the percentage is 14- 20% year round and about 10% on contest day.

After the competition, some bodybuilders have to take an IV to replenish the fluid and nutrients they are lacking!

Something similar occurs with fitness models and photo-shoots:

Several weeks before the big day, they diet in a similar manner as bodybuilders. They cut back their caloric intake so they look their "best."

After the show or shoot, they resume their normal eating habits.

There are several things I want to point out:

1. How a bodybuilder, high end fashion model or runway model looks on the day of the contest or photo shoot is NOT necessarily how they look year round, nor do they eat that way year round.

2. On average, our bodies aren't designed to be in that type of shape all the time. Some people have perfected achieving a "ripped" or "chiseled" look for a specific date or event to a tee.

3. The majority of pictures in magazines are photoshopped. (This will be discussed in detail in another section.) So not only are these models doing extreme diets to get in that shape, their pictures are STILL altered even more.

4. Many models smoke cigarettes to maintain their weight. It is estimated that 13% of women smoke to lose weight, while teenage girls often begin smoking to avoid weight gain.

To make a long story short, the physical looks of some of the individuals you want to look like or emulate may not be all they're cracked up to be.

Our society has tricked us into believing that physical fitness has only one certain look, and if you don't fit this criteria, you're not as in good of shape as you could be, or should be. However, nothing could be further from the truth. There are MANY factors involved.

How many 40 and 50-year-olds do you know who have the body of 20 year old fitness models and bodybuilders with big, strong muscles and sculpted abs?

As we age, our bodies start to change. Our metabolism slows down a bit and our body fat percentages start to increase.

For example, the average body fat percentage for an athletic 20-year-old male is 8-19%, while the percentage for an athletic 50-year-old is 11-22%.

It's extremely difficult (if not downright impossible) for most 50-year-old people to have the body and look of a 20-year-old. Our bodies change over time and it's perfectly natural.

Another important point is that there are different body types: ectomorph, endomorph, and mesomorph. In other words, some people are naturally thin, others are thicker, and others "average."

For example, the big offensive linemen in football are endomorphs.

What about the world class marathon runners? Many of them are very slim in stature and look like they barely weigh 120 pounds. They are ectomorphs: lean with a very fast metabolism.

This is just a really simple example of two very different body types, but in both cases, they are finely tuned athletes.

World class marathon runners are FAST! They can run UNDER 5 minute miles for 2 hours straight. How's that for fitness?

These finely tuned athletes are EXTREMELY fit, but they don't have the "look" that many associate with fitness. Some may even consider them "too skinny."

The NFL linemen are bigger than the average person and may not fit the "fitness standard," but they are VERY strong and a lot faster and nimble than they look!

There are many others, and like these two examples, they probably don't measure up to what society says fitness should LOOK LIKE.

They're fit, but they aren't fitness MODELS.

This is a very important concept to understand and accept as truth: Fitness does NOT have a certain look. Instead of trying to LOOK fit, focus on doing things that will MAKE you fit.

Smoking may help a person lose weight or keep the weight off, but there are plenty of studies out there suggesting a person should NOT smoke.

Starving yourself might help you lose weight, but you also run the risk of missing out on getting enough vitamins and minerals crucial to day-to-day functioning.

How can a person be the best they can be if they are starving themselves?

Instead of watching every calorie, eat the foods that will HELP you become the best person you can be.

Then there's one thing people should take note of, and that's the mentality of most athletes:

"Athletes eat and train, they don't diet and exercise."

Not counting bodybuilders, athletes are trying to be the best athletes they can be, and know that they need to eat the right foods to stay energized and able to complete their workouts.

That means they eat constantly to ensure they get all the nutrients they need.

They aren't trying to starve themselves to get a 6 pack; they are eating a lot, and even if they don't have 6 packs, they are nicely toned.

Now, not all athletes have perfect bodies; but a "perfect body" is NOT needed to be the best you can be.

Just because a person LOOKS like they're in tip top shape doesn't mean they are.

Instead of trying to look athletic, do what athletes do. Change your mindset. Change how you look at workouts and eating. Food is your friend, not something to be avoided.

The right foods, that is!

Athletes understand that in order to get where they want to be, starving themselves will only hurt them, not help them.

Here's an example: The Tour de France is a bike race that lasts 3 weeks. These guys ride, on average, 100 miles a day over all types of terrain: rolling hills, mountains, flatlands, and in all types of weather conditions. They're not just riding, they're RACING, going as fast as they can, riding 4 hours or more a day, every day.

Now, in order for these guys to perform at their best, they eat. A LOT! They understand how important food is to keep their energy levels high enough for this very intense race.

It is suggested that the average person eat 2,000 calories a day to function properly. How much do you think a cyclist riding in the Tour eats?

Tour de France cyclists need to eat up to 9,000 calories a day to maintain their health and weight during the race. Many teams also hire chefs to elevate the meals to gourmet status.

That's a lot of food! But they understand the importance of eating, and eating the right foods for fuel!

And if you look at the average cyclist, they are pretty skinny, even though they eat so much during those three weeks.

The 2005 Tour de France started with 189 starters, with an average height of 5 feet 10.4 inches and weight of 156.2 pounds.

They eat a tremendous amount of food and it is all converted into energy.

Now, I'm NOT saying eat 9,000 calories a day, but eat a good amount of healthy foods that will keep you energized and healthy so you can perform at your best.

The point I'm trying to makes is this: Looking fit and being fit are NOT the same. Don't try look fit by starving yourself. BE fit by working out and training like an athlete. Focus on improving your performance, and your body will improve accordingly. It will happen automatically without you trying.

Fitness comes in all shapes and sizes. Here's a brief list of extremely successful athletes and their measurements:

Usain Bolt. Track & field:
Height: 6' 5" (1.95 m)
Weight: 207 lbs. (94 kg)

Serena Williams. Pro tennis player:
Height: 5' 9" (1.75 m)
Weight: 150 lbs. (68.2 kg)

Derek Jeter. Pro baseball player:
Height: 6' 3" (1.90 m)
Weight: 195 lbs. (88 kg)

Jonathan Quick. Pro hockey player:
Height: 6' 1" (1.85 m)
Weight: 220 lbs. (100 kg)

Gabby Douglas. Gymnast:
Height: 4' 11" (1.50 m)

Weight: 90 lbs. (41 kg)

Alberto Contador. Pro cyclist:
Height: 5' 9" (1.76 m)
Weight: 137 lbs. (62 kg)

Kerri Walsh Jennings. Pro volleyball player:
Height: 6' 2" (1.88 m)
Weight: 157 lbs. (71 kg)

Michael Phelps. World class swimmer:
Height: 6'3" (1.93 m)
Weight: 196 lbs. (89 kg)

LeBron James. Pro basketball player:
Height: 6' 7" (2. 03 m)
Weight: 250 lbs. (113 kg)

Shelly-Ann Fraser-Pryce. Olympic sprinter:
Height: 5'00" (1.52 m)
Weight: 126 lbs. (57 kg)

Bernard Lagat. World class runner:
Height: 5' 8" (1.73 m)
Weight: 134 lbs. (61 kg)

Peyton Manning. Pro football player:
Height: 6' 5" (1.96 m)
Weight: 230 lbs. (104 kg)

Anna Kournikova. Tennis player:
Height: 5' 8" (1.73 m)
Weight: 123 lbs. (56 kg)

Ray Lewis. Pro football player:
Height: 6' 1" (1.87 m)
Weight: 240 lbs. (109 kg)

Every person listed above is extremely fit and has attained a tremendous level of success.

But is LeBron at 6 feet 7 inches more fit than Alberto Contador, who is a foot shorter and 100 pounds lighter? They are both considered among the best in their respective sports.

Is Serena Williams a better athlete than Shelly Ann Frasier?

Michael Phelps may "look" more fit in some people's opinions than Bernard Lagat, but they are BOTH world class athletes and Olympians.

At 6 feet 4 inches and 315 pounds, Michael Oher is considered "obese" based on BMI measurements. Doctors may suggest he lose weight and "get in shape."

On paper he may not look fit, but not only did he win a SUPER BOWL with the Baltimore Ravens, he can run 40 yards in 5.3 seconds and bench press 225 pounds 21 times.

To be his size and achieve those accomplishments a person MUST be fit.

All of these elite athletes eat and they eat well. They understand that to be at their physical and mental best, they MUST consume enough food to keep their energy levels high.

The foods I'm referring to are fruits, vegetables, water, lean protein, and healthy fats found in fish and nuts.

Chances are very slim someone can get fat by eating an apple or banana when they are hungry, but it's a strong possibility someone could gain weight eating a donut or drinking a large soda every day.

Having a 6 pack is nice, but being healthy, not hungry, and not nutrient deficient is better!

Strive to be the best you can be mentally, physically and spiritually. That includes eating the proper foods to give your body the nutrients it deserves to work efficiently.

Don't neglect what's inside. That 6 pack means NOTHING if you have high blood pressure, gout, or elevated cholesterol levels.

I'm 45 years old, and even though I don't have a 6 pack, I'm just as healthy and in shape as I was 20 years ago, when I DID have a 6 pack. My body has changed over the years, and I've learned to EMBRACE the changes and be the best person I can be WITHOUT starving myself to obtain a certain look. I'm still lifting weights and doing triathlons as I was doing 20 years ago, and I feel great!

Looks may fade, but that doesn't mean your health has to as well! Changing your mindset is crucial to being physically fit, but changing your diet is just as important.

CHAPTER 4: EATING FOR FITNESS

There are quite a few components to being physically fit, and it's important to look at the big picture as you embark on your journey. A very important component of being fit in **all** areas of your life is your diet, and I want to talk briefly about our eating habits.

Many people will take a multivitamin, eat an energy bar, or mix a couple scoops of protein powder with water or milk to meet their nutritional needs.

Now most of these products have been vitamin fortified, but I say it is a mistake to think all your nutritional needs can be met this way, or that this gives you the green light to eat whatever you want.

Is it possible these products aren't as good for you as you think and they cannot compare to eating the foods they are trying to emulate?

Yes, that is very possible and I'll explain why. Let me give you an example:

Let's say for breakfast you decide to eat an energy bar. They go by many names: energy bars, protein bars, nutrition bars, health bars, snack bars, food bars, granola bars, etc. Whatever the name, they all claim to offer a nutritional benefit of some sort.

The problem here is all bars aren't created equal, so it's important to look at the label because it may not be as nutritious as you think.

For example, many energy bars are loaded with sugar or high fructose corn syrup. Did you know the ingredients are listed in the order of large to small? In other words, the first ingredients listed have the highest amount, and the last ingredient listed has the smallest quantity.

So when looking at the label on that energy bar, where does the corn syrup, salt, and sugar appear on that label? The closer they are to the left, the more you want to avoid them.

Another ingredient to look for is Partially-Hydrogenated Oils, also known as trans fats. These fats are man-made and have been associated with numerous health issues.

According to many studies, including The Cardiovascular Health Study in the American Journal of Clinical Nutrition in 2006, and a scientific statement from the American Heart Association nutrition committee also in 2006, trans fats can be hazardous to your health.

The studies link Partially-Hydrogenated Oils to increased cholesterol levels, increased risk of allergies, type 2 diabetes, cancer, and heart disease.

A common reaction to this type of information is, *"All this from eating an energy bar?! Is that possible?"*

Yes, it's very possible.

Now, your next thought may be that you only eat one energy bar a day, or every other day, so it's no big deal. You're right: Ever so often it isn't that big of a deal, but it's important to remember that Partially-Hydrogenated Oils are in quite a few foods we eat.

As a society, we eat too many processed foods and it adds up. Think about it: Over the past week, have you eaten any of the following?

Cakes
Cookies
Donuts
Crackers
French fries
Instant mashed potatoes
Pancakes
Microwave popcorn

This is just a small sample of the many foods and products that contain Partially-Hydrogenated Oils.

So, if you ate an energy bar for breakfast, then went to lunch and got a burger and fries or had soup and crackers, you had some of these oils.

Add in a piece of cake in the afternoon or microwave popcorn and you've had quite a bit that day.

It's important to know what you're eating and how it affects your body.

As you can see, eating an energy bar may not be as good for you as you think, even though it's been fortified with vitamins.

Ask yourself: *How good is it if it has added ingredients to it that do more harm than good?*

Can I be the best person I can be physically, mentally and spiritually if

I'm eating these foods on a daily basis?

It should be noted that not all energy bars are full of artificial ingredients, but it's important to read the label and see what's in them. Now, I must admit that I DO eat energy bars that have only natural ingredients, but ONLY during my outdoor triathlon biking or running workouts that last more than 90 minutes. I don't eat them as a meal replacement or snack. Instead, my main meals are primarily unprocessed foods with a variety of fruits and vegetables daily. Avoid energy bars that have sugar, sodium and artificial flavoring and ingredients as they are nothing more than fancy candy bars!

Even though I do eat energy bars for my extended workouts, my point still stands that it's important to eat natural foods and I'll explain why in the next sections.

HOW GOOD ARE PROTEIN SHAKES?

Protein shakes are widely accepted and very popular. Many people drink the shakes daily, sometimes 2-3 servings within 24 hours.

Even though the shakes are considered safe and an effective weight loss tool, there are some things to keep in mind:

According to some fitness experts and physicians, people get enough protein from their daily diets, and they really don't need the extra protein.

I am 6 feet, 220 pounds. I've been lifting weights for over 25 years and haven't taken protein supplements since I first started, and even then I only did it for several months. I get all my protein from my foods, and lately I've been getting more of it from non-meat sources.

Here's an interesting study by Consumer Reports in 2010:

"We purchased 15 protein powders and drinks mainly in the New York metro area or online and tested multiple samples of each for arsenic,

cadmium, lead, and mercury. The results showed a considerable range, but levels in three products were of particular concern because consuming three servings a day could result in daily exposure to arsenic, cadmium, or lead exceeding the limits proposed by USP."

Arsenic, Cadmium, and Lead.

The question that MUST be asked is WHY are these harmful ingredients being put into something that we eat, let alone something that is supposed to be healthy?

How many people drink these shakes daily?

The report also says:

"When these toxic heavy metals are combined in a product that is marketed for daily use that raises serious public health concerns, especially for pregnant women, children, and young adults."

Just because a product is being advertised as healthy doesn't mean it really is. Being mentally, physically and spiritually fit also means being aware of what you are ingesting and how it can affect you.

Remember: This is YOUR health we're talking about.

Many people do not know cadmium was found in some protein shakes. They also may not realize they are being exposed to it and how it affects their bodies.

Cadmium is of no use to the human body and is toxic, even at low levels. The negative effects of cadmium on the body are numerous and can impact nearly all systems in the body, including cardiovascular, reproductive, the kidneys, eyes, and even the brain.

Cadmium affects blood pressure, prostate function and testosterone levels, induces bone damage, and can affect renal and dopaminergic systems in children.

The point here is that people can have any of these symptoms described and it could be due to the cadmium they have been ingesting day after day, month after month, year after year.

It's very possible a person may have these symptoms and are prescribed medication to help cure them or make them feel better. That's all well and good, but if they don't know that their blood pressure issues were caused by the cadmium in the first place, they might continue with their normal routine, which may include ingesting "healthy" products that are the actual cause of the problem.

So now a person is taking medicine to feel better, but it's all for naught because they are still using the product making them sick in the first place.

A misdiagnosis can be hazardous to your health as well devastating to your bank account.

Now I'm not saying that a protein shake will cause these problems in 100% of people, but it's important to know the possible dangers of using these products.

A knowledgeable consumer is a smart consumer.

Another thing to consider is this:

Federal regulations do not generally require that protein drinks and other dietary supplements be tested before they are sold to ensure that they are safe, effective, and free of contaminants, as the rules require of prescription drugs.

Basically, we have to trust the manufacturer to make sure the product is safe.

So, truth be told, we may not really know what's in these products or what the long term effects are until years later.

I strongly suggest you look into this yourself. Do your own research as to what you're eating and how it can affect you.

Which brings me back to my original point:
Instead of relying on these man-made supplements, eat natural foods to meet your nutritional needs. Try as we might, man can NOT replicate EXACTLY what nature can do.

You may think you're getting the benefits by eating a manmade substitute, but you're not.

Let's say you decide to eat an energy bar in the morning. You look at the label and it has quite a few vitamins and minerals.

Or you make a protein shake, or take a multivitamin and eat a bagel with it.

Now let's compare that to someone eating an apple or banana for breakfast.

1. One benefit of eating apples is that they are called "Nature's Toothbrush."

An apple won't replace your toothbrush, but biting and chewing an apple stimulates the production of saliva in your mouth, reducing tooth decay by lowering the levels of bacteria.

They also help clean plaque from teeth and freshen breath.

That energy bar won't do that. Matter of fact, if it's loaded with sugar it may DAMAGE your teeth.

2. Another benefit is reduced cholesterol. The soluble fiber found in apples binds with fats in the intestine, which translates into lower cholesterol levels and a healthier you.

What energy bar or protein shake out there can reduce cholesterol?

3. Women who eat at least one apple a day are 28% less likely to develop type 2 diabetes than those who don't eat apples. Apples are loaded with soluble fiber, the key to blunting blood sugar swings.

Multivitamins aren't touted as products that can decrease diabetes.

Some of the health benefits you get from food can't be duplicated in a lab.

Let's look at bananas. Bananas can be eaten at any time and are enjoyed by people of all ages. Some of the health benefits of bananas include the following:

Lower blood pressure
Anti-inflammatory
Help maintain regular heartbeat
Ease constipation
Reduce symptoms of nicotine withdrawal
Good food source for those with ulcers
Help curb sugar cravings

And these are just some of the benefits. It's also known that bananas are an excellent source of potassium and vitamin B6.

You would be hard pressed to find a single vitamin that claims to have all these health benefits.

If a person went to a doctor with any of the issues described above like ulcers, constipation, and high blood pressure, they couldn't take just one pill, they would be prescribed several.

Their medicine cabinet would be jam packed with (expensive) pills, and many people's medicine cabinets are.

The drug industry is a multi-billion dollar industry and many people are making a nice living off of your illnesses.

Then there's the dangers of mixing medicines and dangerous side effects.

The point I'm trying to make is that foods can have quite different reactions in the body. Just isolating and extracting the nutrients in foods like what we see in the shakes and the vitamins doesn't always work.

A supplement might only contain vitamin C for example, which may not digest into the cancer-fighting forms without the other components in the real food.

I'm barely scratching the surface here with these examples of apples and bananas, but it's important people understand the significance of eating REAL FOOD. If a person thinks popping a pill or munching an energy bar is going to keep them healthy, they're making a mistake.

The human body is very intricate and the good foods we eat like spinach, tomatoes, grapes, strawberries (and many others) are designed to keep us healthy, but many times we turn on the television and see advertisements about a new drug that is supposed to cure whatever is wrong with us.

In reality, it comes back to the foods we eat. What people tend to forget is some of the junk food we eat is making us sick in the first place.

Eat good food and minimize the junk food you eat on a daily basis and your body's immune system will be strong enough to fight off disease.

Every day, make an effort to eat a variety of fruits and veggies. Eat nuts and raisins for a mid-morning snack. Eat an apple on the way home from work. Have a banana with your breakfast. Decrease the processed foods in your life and your body will thank you!

ENERGY DRINKS: ARE THEY WORTH IT?

It's 3:00 pm. You were feeling good, then all of a sudden, you hit a brick wall! You have two more hours to go before you can head home, but all of a sudden, you can barely keep your eyes open.

You have a meeting in five minutes or you have to work on an important project. You have a deadline to meet, but all you want to do is go to your car and take a nap!

You need a pick-me-up—fast! What to do, what to do?

Drink a soda?

Grab a candy bar?
No, wait! How about an energy drink!

You try and it really peps you up within minutes. You're excited and feeling good! You feel like you're on top of the world and ready for anything!

You start to take them on a regular basis, any time you need a pick-me-up.

Sound familiar?

What are these magical drinks? Are they good for me? How do they affect me physically? Mentally? Before we analyze the drinks, take a step back and ask yourself:

WHY do I get tired and sluggish in the first place?

Is there something I can do to prevent myself from getting tired?

Are there alternatives to energy drinks and junk food?

When trying to be the best you can be, it's important to LISTEN TO YOUR BODY. Your body is ALWAYS talking to you. It's very vocal! Sometimes it's very loud.

If you're hungry, your body tells you.

If you stub your toe at 2 am while going to the bathroom, it tells you it's in pain.

If you're too hot or too cold, it lets you know.

It even lets you know when it's under stress. You just have to listen to it.

The afternoon sluggish or sleepy feeling could be caused by many things. The key here is to do an "internal investigation."

Are you not getting enough rest at night?

Is it something you ate at lunch that's making you sluggish?

Are you simply bored or not mentally stimulated?

Each of these can be rectified without taking an energy drink or eating junk, but let's look at each of these:

Sleep: If you don't get enough rest, you'll feel sluggish. A sluggish body = a slower metabolism. Slower metabolism = weight gain.

So if you're indeed not getting enough rest, it's possible you're eating a high calorie snack like a chocolate bar or a soda to give you that extra boost of energy.

Yes, you're getting that boost of energy, but you're also getting extra calories that you're NOT burning off. These calories will add up and turn into extra pounds as time goes on.

The average adult needs 7-9 hours of sleep per night. How many are you getting?

Sluggish after lunch: If we eat a heavy meal, many of us will feel very sluggish and sleepy shortly thereafter. One reason is it can be related to eating processed foods that contain high levels of sugar and refined carbohydrates. Eating these types of foods causes a rise in blood sugar levels, followed by a drop, which results in low energy levels or the "crash."

Eating smaller, more frequent meals can help alleviate this sluggish feeling, as this will keep your energy levels high. Aim for 5-6 small meals per day.

Another possible reason could be due to food allergies or intolerances, which are usually associated with digestive problems such as indigestion, bloating, constipation, gas, or diarrhea.

This is when listening to your body is key. Try and remove certain foods from your diet for two weeks, then slowly reintroduce them one by one. If you notice any changes, you might have a food allergy. This could be the cause of your sluggishness.

Boredom: There's nothing worse than sitting in a boring class or meeting. The topic doesn't interest you and you can't escape. Meetings right after lunch can be a nightmare!

This is a tricky one to fix if you're in a controlled setting. While it's important to pay attention, doing something that will keep you mentally stimulated will keep you awake. Try taking notes with your opposite hand; munch on fruit instead of candy to keep your blood sugar levels high; ask questions; or take a short walk several minutes before the meeting to energize you.

These are some natural, healthier ways to keep awake, but many times, we prefer to use artificial, man-made products that are meant to wake us up or make us alert. One of those products is energy drinks.

The Energy Drink market is a billion dollar industry. It is projected that annual sales will reach $21 billion by 2017.

While the energy drinks and shots market may be a small component of the non-alcoholic beverage industry, it is moving up rapidly, growing 60% from 2008-2012 according to Packaged Facts estimates in an all-new research report, "Energy Drinks and Shots: U.S. Market Trends." In 2012, total U.S. sales for the energy drinks and shots market was worth more than $12.5 billion.

A lot of money is being made, and a lot of these drinks are being consumed, but at what price? Sure, they may wake us up, but how many calories of this product are we consuming? How many grams of sugar do these products have? How safe are these products? Where did they come from?

Let's examine the energy drinks market:

Energy drinks have been around for decades, with the first widely known energy drink being Coca-Cola in 1904. It was made with two know stimulants (cocoa leaves and kola nuts) and was originally marketed as an energy booster. These stimulants are in essence cocaine. (Of course the Coke we drink today does not have cocaine in its ingredients.)

Joining the world of energy drinks are still the popular brands: Bacchus-F and Lipovitan. From Korea and Japan respectively, these are more akin to the modern 5-Hour Energy. They come in small bottles, designed to be taken whole or in halves as a nutritional supplement.

Bacchus-F was created in the 1960s and is available in the United States and Singapore.

Energy drinks contain about three times the amount of caffeine as cola. Twelve ounces of Coca-Cola Classic contains 35 mg of caffeine, whereas a Monster Energy Drink contains 120 mg of caffeine.

Currently, the amount of caffeine added to energy drinks is not regulated by the FDA, so often the amounts listed (if they're listed) may not be accurate.

A study published in the Journal of Pediatrics reports that more teens are drinking energy drinks. In 2003, 16% regularly consumed the drinks, while in 2008, that percentage jumped to 35%.

One study of college student consumption found 50% of students drank at least one to four a month. This year, research documented a jump in energy drink-related emergency room visits and politicians and consumers called upon the Food and Drug Administration (FDA) to look into deaths associated with the drinks.

As of 2013, in the United States some energy drinks, including Monster Energy and Rockstar Energy, were reported to be rebranding their products as beverages rather than as dietary supplements. As beverages, they would be relieved of FDA reporting requirements with respect to deaths and injuries and can be purchased with food stamps, but must list ingredients on the can.

There is no official recommended limit for the amount of caffeine a person can consume, but excessive caffeine has been linked to a variety of adverse effects such as high blood pressure, premature birth and possibly sudden death.

Also, the sugar content in energy drinks ranges from 21 grams to 34 grams per 8 ounces, and can come in the form of sucrose, glucose, or high fructose corn syrup.

Also according to the Journal of Pediatrics, "Users who consume two or three energy drinks could be taking in 120 mg to 180 mg of sugar, which is 4 to 6 times the maximum recommended daily intake," the authors write, noting that adolescents who consume energy drinks could be at risk for obesity and dental problems.

So, are energy drinks bad for you? It depends on who you ask.

Some studies show energy drinks reported significant improvements in mental and cognitive performances as well as increased subjective alertness.

On the flip side, in the US, energy drinks have been linked with reports of nausea, abnormal heart rhythms and emergency room visits. The drinks may cause seizures due to the "crash" following the energy high that occurs after consumption. Caffeine dosage is not required to be on the product label for food in the United States, unlike drugs, but some advocates are urging the FDA to change this practice.

It may be years before we know the full effects of energy drinks as the long term effects have yet to be realized. These drinks have high amounts of caffeine and there are many studies that show how addictive caffeine can be.

In order to be the best you can be physically, it's crucial to become in tune with your body. Looking for the "quick fix" doesn't solve the problem. In this case, it could actually cause other problems, such as becoming addicted to caffeine or possibly experiencing side effects from drinking too many of these energy drinks.

The question you must keep asking yourself is WHY do you need the energy drink in the first place?

Energy drinks are a quick fix. They'll give you energy for a brief moment, but may not be best for long term use. Don't rely on these for your energy levels. Instead, LISTEN TO YOUR BODY. The energy drink will help short term, but it's not a long term solution.

CHAPTER 5: WHAT'S YOUR BODY TYPE?

As you can see, being physically fit is more than just physical exercise. It's just as important to be fit on the inside as well as the outside.

In the previous section, we discussed how *looking fit* and *being fit* are two different things. We also talked about the importance of eating whole foods as opposed to taking supplements and energy drinks. A person can understand that concept, but they still may not be satisfied with how they look. A key aspect of being physically and MENTALLY fit is being comfortable with yourself and your appearance. Being the best YOU can be and being perfect are two totally different things. It's important to exercise and live a healthy lifestyle, but it's also important to know what your limitations are and to be realistic.

For example, a person who is 5'2" but wants to be taller shouldn't obsess over this or feel they are less than the person who is their ideal height.

Instead on dwelling on something that's out of your control, try to be the best 5'2" person YOU can be!

Then we have issues with body types and body images. Many will obsess about having a certain look or body type. Some women may feel less of a person because they don't have an hourglass figure and some men aren't happy because they don't have large muscles, broad shoulders and a narrow waist.

There's nothing wrong with aspiring to look a certain way, but it's also important to be realistic.

When wanting to make changes with your appearance, there are several things that must be taken into account:

Age: How old are you? The older you are, the more difficult it will be to achieve the look you want. Our metabolism slows down as we age. Our muscle mass decreases. These changes are amplified if you haven't taken care of your body.

Mind you, this does NOT mean to simply give up and not try! Exercise is great for those of all ages and physical conditions. The key is to go into an exercise program with realistic expectations so you won't get discouraged and give up.

With that being said, there are other factors to consider when wanting to make changes.

Body type: There are 3 body types, and your body type will play a large part in your physical look:

Ectomorph

Ectomorphs have slim bones, long limbs, very little body fat and very little muscle. Ballerinas, supermodels and basketball players often fall into this group due to their delicately built frames. Bruce Lee, Kevin Durant, Cameron Diaz and Chris Rock are examples of ectomorphs.

Endomorph

Endomorphs have round, soft and curvy bodies, having the opposite characteristics of the ectomorphs. They have slow metabolisms, gain fat easily and have a hard time losing weight. They often have large frames, with hips that tend to be wider than their shoulders by a fair bit, creating a pear-shaped physique. John Goodman, Oprah Winfrey, Danny DeVito, and Queen Latifah are classic endomorphs.

Mesomorph

Mesomorphs are characterized as athletic, strong, compact, and naturally lean with excellent posture. Often, their shoulders are wider than their hips. Mesomorphs are natural athletes and tend to be lean and muscular without trying, known for having a "medium" build. Angela Bassett, Arnold Schwarzenegger, and Anna Kournikova are classic mesomorphs.

Below is a chart showing the different body types side by side.

Ectomorph	Endomorph	Mesomorph
Typically skinny	Soft, round body	Hourglass shape (women) Hard, muscular body (men)
Slim/Slender Stature	Underdeveloped muscles	Naturally Lean/athletic
Lower body fat %	Higher Body fat %	Body fat evenly distributed
Fast metabolism	Slow metabolism	Loses fat easily

Difficulty Gaining Weight	Gains weight easily	Gains or loses weight easily
Difficulty Gaining Muscle	Gains muscle easily	Gains muscle quickly
Small joints	Medium/large joints	Medium sized joints

What's important to consider here is your metabolism. Each body type has its specific characteristics when it comes to burning calories and losing weight.

Ectomorphs tend to have trouble gaining weight no matter how much they eat.

Mesomorphs can lose weight quickly through diet and exercise.

An endomorph has trouble losing weight and it takes them a little longer to do so.

Knowing your body type will help you keep things in perspective when it comes to reaching your fitness goals.

If your best friend is an ectomorph and you are an endomorph, don't be surprised (or upset) if she sees results faster than you, even though you're doing the same workout.

It's also important to be realistic: a male endomorph who is 5'9", 220 lbs. probably can't look like a 5'11", 175 lbs. mesomorph or 6'2", 165 lbs. ectomorph. On the flip side, it'll be difficult for that ectomorph to have the look of that mesomorph. Difficult? Yes. Impossible? No.

It's important to accept yourself for who you are. None of us are perfect. We've ALL had things about ourselves that we'd like to change at some point in our lives.

Instead of dwelling on our imperfections or looking at others and wishing we have what they have, be PROUD of what you DO have. Embrace your individuality. Unless you have an identical twin, there's no one out there like you. Be proud of what you DO have!

But at the same time, work on being the best person YOU can be, and that includes following the philosophies in this book.

It's also important to find exercises that are suited for you and your body type, not what's in style today, or what your best friend is doing. Just because it's popular doesn't mean that's what's right for YOU.

So what are you: ecto, endo, or meso? Knowing your body type will help you strive for a more realistic goal. Not only that, knowing up front what you are will help prevent frustration as you embark on your fitness journey. Here are some suggested exercises based on your body type.

Ectomorph. The average ectomorph wants to get bigger. They are relatively slim even though they can consume a lot of calories daily.

Weight training is key for ectomorphs, but it must be done properly. It's easy for them to over train because they have high energy levels. Sessions should be 3 days per week, with a rest day in between. Resting approximately 2-3 minutes between sets is advised.

Many ectomorphs are new to weight training, so basic exercises are fine as their bodies adjust to rigors of the activity. A "pyramid routine" will help them get the right mix of intensity and frequency. Too much intensity and they run the risk of overtraining. For each exercise perform 3-4 sets with a rep scheme of 10-8-6-15.

- Bench Press (Barbell or Dumbbell)

- Seated Lateral Raises

- Barbell Bent over rows

- Seated Shoulder presses (Barbell or dumbbell)

- Bicep curls (curl bar, straight bar or dumbbells)

- Triceps extension (lying or standing)

- Squats

Most male ectomorphs want to gain weight while some female ecto's simply want to tone and shape. For those women who want to tone, they can forgo the pyramid and simply perform 12-15 reps of each exercise described above.

Cardio: When I graduated high school in 1986 I was 5'10," 135 pounds. A classic ectomorph. Today, I'm a 6'00," 225 pounds mesomorph, but I can still do the cardio I did while in high school, and then some. I grew up doing cardio then stopped for a year in 1987 to concentrate on weight training. After one year started doing cardio again. I still gained muscle mass as I was performing a routine similar to the one above.

I bring this up because many will advise ectomorphs to cut back on the cardio or stop altogether. While the ectomorph's goal is to gain mass, the goal of this book is to be the best you can be, and that includes having strength *and* cardiovascular fitness. Weight training can be your primary goal, but don't neglect cardio. Aim for 30 minutes of cardio a minimum of two times a week. The cardio can be whatever you choose: walking, jogging, swimming, basketball, etc. Whatever it is, make sure it's something you enjoy!

Diet: If an ectomorph wants to gain weight, they have to take in more calories than they burn. That's the short and simple answer but it's not so easy for ectomorphs. They should eat 5-8 times per day. Breakfast, lunch, and dinner should be full, hearty meals with two or more snacks in between. These should be foods they enjoy, because not many of us can eat a lot of something we don't like. Even though the goal is to gain weight, the foods should be healthy foods. Keep junk foods, sodas, and processed foods to a minimum.

Keep in mind it could take years before the ectomorph reaches their desired weight and size. That means they will have been eating a lot of food on a regular basis for a very long time. If they keep the same eating habits after they've reached their goal, they will continue to gain weight. This must be kept in mind and diets should be modified accordingly if this situation arises.

An ideal diet for ectomorphs would be 55% carbs, 25% protein, and 20% fat. Here's a breakdown on the food types:

Carbohydrates. Not all carbohydrates are created equal. Healthy carbs for are fruits, vegetables, and whole grains like rice, whole grain breads, quinoa, amaranth, millet, corn, barley, dried fruits, yams, and sweet potatoes. Avoid the empty carbs like processed foods, cakes, cookies, potato chips and other sweets.

Protein. Avoid the high fat proteins found in fast food and fried food. Instead, eat lean protein such as fish, poultry, beans, tofu, lean beef and egg whites.

Fats. Like carbs, not all fats are created equal. Good fats are essential for maintaining healthy skin, and it plays a central role in promoting proper eyesight and brain development in babies and children. It is a major source of energy and helps absorb some vitamins and minerals. It is essential for blood clotting, muscle movement, and inflammation. These are the good fats, which include monounsaturated and polyunsaturated fats, which many of us don't get enough of. These would include nuts, seeds, oily fish, avocados, and oils such as olive oil, peanut oil, canola oil, as well as high-oleic safflower and sunflower oils.

These types of fats should be eaten daily by all body types.

Bad fats include industrial-made trans fats. Saturated fats fall somewhere in the middle. Many of us eat too many trans fats and not enough monounsaturated and polyunsaturated fats. Eating foods rich in trans fats increases the amount of harmful LDL cholesterol in the bloodstream and reduces the amount of beneficial HDL cholesterol. Many fast foods and processed foods fall into this category and should be avoided.

Endomorph. Since endomorphs tend to have a harder time losing weight than other body types, it is suggested they weight train 3-4 times a week and do cardio 2-3 times a week. The reason being is the increased muscle mass will also increase their basal metabolic rate, or BMR. The BMR is defined as the minimum number of calories needed to support basic functions, including breathing and circulation.

Exactly how much of an increase this will generate has been debated many times over the years and is still ongoing. As of this writing, the general consensus is that a pound of muscle at rest burns about six calories per day and a pound of fat burns about two. That may not sound like much, but if a person weighs 250-300 pounds or more, the increased BMR could be significant.

Endomorphs should focus on exercises that work several muscles at once with 30-60 seconds rest between sets. This routine is suitable for both men and women:

- Chest: Bench presses with a barbell or dumb bell (incline, decline, or flat bench.)

- Back: Deadlifts, bent-over rows,

- Shoulders: Military press, dumb bell overhead press

- Legs: Squats, leg presses, lunges

- Abs: Planks, Leg Raises

- Cardio: Swimming, brisk walking, cycling or any activity they enjoy that can be done without causing any strain or injury (with a doctor's approval.)

Don't have access to a gym or don't like to lift weights? Bodyweight exercises are just as effective. Pushups, lunges, squats, and planks are great bodyweight exercises that target all the major muscle groups.

Diet. Since endomorph's have slow metabolisms, it's important they eat foods that are healthy and nutritious. Junk food is the last thing they need as it tends to pack on the pounds.

An ideal diet for endomorphs to eat 5-6 smaller meals per day, with a mix of 25% carbs, 35% protein, and 40% fat.

Other helpful tips for endomorphs is to get adequate sleep nightly and to spend less time doing sedentary activities like watching television.

Mesomorph. Mesomorphs are the most popular body type. They are glamorized in movies and in magazines. They also have the most freedom as far as working out because they tend to see positive results in anything they do. With that said, there are some things they can do to get the most out of their workouts.

Some female mesomorphs may be resistant to weight training because they don't want to get too bulky. Lifting light to moderate weights 2-3 times a week will help shape and tone as opposed to becoming big and bulky. Female mesomorphs should aim for 2 to 3 sets of 10 – 12 repetitions using light to moderate weights for each major muscle group.

Male mesomorphs need to lift moderate to heavy weights to stimulate muscle growth. A moderate routine would be 3 to 4 exercises for each muscle group, with 3-4 sets per exercise. Each set can consist of 12-15 repetitions. A heavy lifting program consists of 3-4 sets of 6-8 reps with increasing weight load each set.

The average mesomorph (male or female) adapts quickly to exercises and need to change their strength training routines often. Mesomorphs can perform a wide variety of exercises with few limitations. They can perform the exercises described for the other body types as well as more advanced programs.

Diet. Even though mesomorphs have what some describe as the "perfect body," that doesn't mean they can eat whatever they want. They must eat a balanced diet to keep their physiques.

Like the others, mesomorphs should eat healthy meals frequently throughout the day. While ectomorphs may eat 5-8 meals, mesomorphs can eat 5-6 (three main meals and two to three snacks.) A balanced diet is best, eating complex carbohydrates like fruits and veggies, lean proteins, and healthy fats.

An ideal diet for mesomorphs would consist of 40% carbohydrate, 30% protein, and 30% fat.

Please note: The primary goal is to be healthy, so if you prefer to do a certain exercise or activity, by all means continue to do that. The above exercises are merely suggestions and not set in stone. However, it's also important to know your limitations and what exercises may do more harm than good.

For example, if you're extremely obese, jogging or running may put too much pressure on your knees and possibly cause injuries.

While everyone around you is running, walking, swimming, or jogging in water may be better suited for you.

On the other hand, if an ectomorph wants to gain weight, high intensity cardio may not be their best option. He may want to go walking with an endomorph. Even though they are walking together, they are doing it for different reasons.

Keep all these factors in mind the next time you see a product that guarantees weight loss, before and after photos, or when you participate in a group fitness class. Not everyone will have the same results!

It's also important to note that some people are a combination of body types. Some may even change body types over time as I did. These are factors that should not be overlooked.

Here's another handy chart comparing male body types and ways to train them as described above. (Seeing them side by side may help put things in perspective.) The ectomorph wants to gain weight, the endomorph wants to lose weight, and the mesomorph is content the way he is:

	Ectomorph	Endomorph	Mesomorph
Diet	55% carbs	25% carbs	40% carbs
	25% protein	35% protein	30% protein
	20% fat	40% fat	30% fat
Strength	3x/week	4x/week	3x/week
Training	3-4 sets	3-4 sets	3-4 sets
	Pyramid reps	8-10 reps	6-8 reps
Cardio	1-2x per week	2-3x per week	3x per week

In addition to body types, it's important to know if you have any health issues or injuries. In other words, certain exercises are to be avoided if you have a medical condition:

High blood pressure: It is advised that people with high blood pressure avoid exercises that cause them to bend over for extended periods of time (i.e. the yoga move, Downward Dog).

Diabetes: Diabetics may be advised to avoid activities that involve strenuous lifting, high-impact activities like running, or placing the head in an inverted position for extended periods of time like the Downward Dog.

Kidney disease: Strenuous exercises including weight training should be avoided.

This is just a small sample of things that must be taken into account when starting an exercise program. There are many other illnesses out there and it's up to you to learn not only what may be wrong with you, but what exercises should be avoided.

No matter your physical condition, it is STRONGLY advised you have a physical before you begin an exercise routine. A person may not know something is wrong with them, and even though their heart is in the right place, the wrong exercise could be dangerous for them.

Remember: Just because an exercise is popular doesn't mean it's right for YOU. Listen to your body. Learn what your strengths and weaknesses are and work on you. Don't worry what everyone is doing!

When a person recognizes their body type and has determined what exercises work best for their particular goals, they can begin to focus and work hard to get where they want to be.

CHAPTER 6: IMPROVING YOUR FAST & SLOW TWITCH MUSCLES

Many of you reading this may be wondering what I consider to be the best exercises or routines a person should do. It's extremely easy for me to say, *Jog for 30 minutes a day, 3 times a week and hold a plank for 2 minutes every day.* While that may be an effective exercise program, if a person isn't taking other variables into account (such as their body type or fitness goal,) it might not be the best program for them.

For example, if a person just had a knee or hip replacement, that advice is not going to help them. What if a person simply doesn't LIKE to run? The above advice will fall on deaf ears in both instances. I always ask my clients what exercises they like, because if they like it, they are more apt to do it and stick with it.

The purpose here is to give a person the tools to find the right exercises for them based on their own unique situation. It's also important to recognize habits and activities they may be currently doing that are keeping them from reaching their fitness goals. One such factor is what we will discuss now.

Do you know anyone who is a great distance runner, but a slow sprinter? Ever wonder how some people can jump extremely high while others can ride a bike for hours and hours and not get tired? The answer lies in the muscles.

In the simplest of terms, our bodies are composed of two types of muscle fibers: slow twitch fibers (Type I) and fast twitch muscle fibers (Type II).

Fast twitch fibers are used for fast, explosive movements like sprinting, jumping, and throwing a fast boxing jab or kick. These muscles are used for a short period of time and fatigue quickly. (This is why you see people breathing hard after a 100 or 200 yard dash.) Slow twitch fibers are used for long endurance activities like marathons and triathlons. Even in endurance events, fast twitch fibers can be useful if a person needs to sprint or increase speed significantly for a short period of time.

The average person has 50% fast twitch fibers and 50% slow twitch fibers in their muscles, but that may vary among elite athletes. For example, world class sprinters like Usain Bolt may have 80% fast twitch muscle fibers in their thighs, while a cyclist like Alberto Contador may have 80% slow twitch fibers in the same muscle groups.

It is said that variety is the spice of life. That can also be applied to exercising. Go to any gym in America and you will see people walking, jogging, using the stair master, or riding the stationary bike at a slow speed for an extended period of time. The fact they are exercising is to be applauded, but since we all have both fast and slow twitch muscle fibers in our bodies, why not work both types of muscles?

Fast Twitch Training

Want explosive speed, strength and power? If you do, fast twitch training is needed. (If you're attacked by someone and need to defend yourself that fast, explosive power would come in handy!) Here are some exercises to build your fast twitch muscle fibers:

1. Lift weights. Lifting heavy weights will make you stronger and trigger your fast twitch fibers and power.

2. Sprints. Run for 30-50 yards as hard and as fast as you can. Walk for a minute and repeat. Do this 5 times.

3. Plyometric Exercises. Hopping up on a bench, jumps, and leaps are great for explosive strength.

4. Eat protein. Protein intake is needed to encourage muscle healing and growth. It is very difficult to recover from sprint workouts without eating enough protein. Fish, chicken, turkey, nuts and lean beef are excellent sources.

5. Intervals. While riding the stationary bike, walking or jogging, create a program where you go as fast as you can for 10-60 seconds, then slow down and resume your original pace.

Slow Twitch Training

Athletes who run marathons, compete in triathlons and can ride a bike for hours at a time have well developed slow twitch muscle fibers. We all have the ability to perform these feats. It's just a matter of training these muscles.

Building slow twitch fibers is relatively simple. These muscles are very efficient and designed for endurance. The key is to get out there and use them: Go for a walk, a slow jog, bike ride, or swim. As time goes on, gradually increase your distances. Your muscles will adapt and eventually you'll be able to increase your speed and intensity as well as the distance. Patience is the key here because it takes time to build your endurance.

In time, you'll be able to go further than you ever imagined because the human body is capable of accomplishing amazing feats. Gladys Burril completed a marathon at 92 years old, making her the oldest marathon finisher. If she can develop her slow twitch muscles well enough to complete a marathon then we can too!

Ever see what happens to a car that sits without being driven? It starts to look run down and when you try to start it, it won't crank. It needs a jump start. The same thing happens to our muscles: They start to lose their muscle tone, and when you try to use them like you did 20 years ago, they won't respond. Your muscles will need a jump start just like that car. The key is to not let your muscles "sit." Stay active and incorporate a variety of exercises in your routine that use both slow and fast twitch muscles.

Training both your fast twitch and slow twitch muscles will help you become a better-rounded athlete. It is also a great way to mix up your workouts and can be an effective cross training tool as well, which is discussed in the next chapter.

CHAPTER 7: THE BENEFITS OF CROSS TRAINING

The information in the previous sections is designed to help you become more informed about the choices you make and how foods and supplements can affect you. As you can see, there's more to reaching your full potential than just working out. What you're doing when you're NOT working out is just as important for your physical health (if not more). It's these other factors that can make or break you, and we are slowly putting the pieces of the puzzle together.

Now, I won't tell you what the best exercises are to do for 30 minutes (or more), as each of us will have our own preferences. But what I WILL suggest is choosing several exercises, and I will explain why.

Many of you know I do triathlons. I really enjoy doing these races because they push me to my physical and mental limits. It's the ultimate challenge to perform in three separate sports on the same day.

My start in triathlon was purely by accident. In high school I ran track and cross country, but once I graduated I stopped running and focused on lifting weights, and that's all I did.

One day, I was lifting weights and my mother blurted out: *"All you do is lift weights. You need to run around that track!"*

We lived across the street from a high school that had a 400 meter track.

To be honest, I didn't want to do any cardio because I wanted to gain weight. I thought doing the cardio would hurt me. But I respected what my mother said and decided to jog once a week to keep the peace.

Needless to say, I rediscovered my passion for running and started running more and more.

I did some research and learned about the importance of doing cardio, and that most pro bodybuilders did some sort of cardio.

I was under the impression that a thin person, as I was at the time, should stay away from cardio, as that would prevent me from gaining any weight or muscle mass.

That's not necessarily true, because many track and field athletes (especially the sprinters) are well built and muscular. Same with many pro football running backs. They each do a tremendous amount of cardio yet are still big and strong.

Once I obtained this information, I started to change my mindset about fitness: I wanted to have a good combination of strength AND endurance. I wanted to be as comfortable in the weight room with big bodybuilders as I was with distance runners.

Why not have the best of both worlds?

It was around this time frame that a friend and I came up with the idea to become lifeguards.

This was perfect timing as I was really getting into the fitness lifestyle. What better way to get in better shape AND get paid at the same time?

I remained a lifeguard for several years, working at various hotels and condominiums in the Chicago area. Being a guard was great because it forced me to keep swimming to stay in shape, thus helping with my cross training.

Years later, that swimming background helped me muster up the courage to try my first triathlon and the rest, as they say, is history!

Coming from an athletic background, my transition into cross training was a gradual one, but I think everyone should find AT LEAST two activities they enjoy.

One great reason is to prevent boredom or monotony. Some people enjoy doing the same activity over and over, but this isn't the best approach to fitness. In time, your body gets used to that exercise and will become more efficient at it. The more efficient it is, the less energy it has to put out.

Think of it another way. If a person is cross country skiing, which would take more energy: a person following the ski tracks of the people who rode that course before them or a person who's skiing over snow that no one has skied on before?

Or if a person is walking through the jungle, who is using more energy: the person with a sickle carving out his own path or the person following the path already made?

In both cases, your body creates its own "path" in time, making it easier and easier for future workouts.

In order to reap the same benefits from the workout, a person should increase the intensity or make some other changes. For some, this is a problem because they are hesitant to push themselves. We've all seen the person on the stair master or stationary bike moving at a slow pace day after day, month after month. We also see them looking the exact same day after day, month after month.

Some exercise is better than none at all, but if a person is just going through the motions, they cannot expect to be the best they can be nor should they expect to get the body they *think* they deserve.

Pushing yourself requires you to get out of your comfort zone, and basically that means being uncomfortable for a while. Our society has spoiled us into expecting results pretty easily and with minimal effort, but when it comes to your health and fitness levels, there are no shortcuts.

You have no choice but to push yourself. Not only that, increase the VARIETY of exercises you do to reap the most benefits.

Let's use runners as an example.

They really enjoy running and have been doing it for several years. They have ran in a couple 5k's and even in a half marathon. Their goal next year is to run in a full marathon.

They LOVE to run and get the "runner's high" quite often. When they run, they are leaving all their problems and stress on the jogging path and feel like a new person when they're finished. They feel renewed and ready to take on the world.

This example is quite real. Many runners can attest to that feeling when running, especially outdoors in the fresh air.

I've experienced it many times and it's like a feeling of euphoria. You become totally in tune with your body and you feel as if you're floating, not running. Your energy feels unlimited, your mind is totally clear and at peace. It's a wonderful feeling!

Many runners can also attest to striving to get better and participating in races, trying to improve their times.

This is great, as the person in this example is reaping the benefits of exercise and is steadily improving by increasing the intensity of their workout.

If that's the case, what's the problem?

Well, in this case, running is all they truly enjoy. No other activity gives them that runner's high or relieves their stress like running does. Since this is all they do, other muscles in their body aren't getting worked. Their upper body isn't as finely conditioned as their lower body.

Their hamstrings aren't as developed as their thighs.

Then there's the possibility of injury due to over use. Common injuries for runners are:

Shin splints
Knee problems (runner's knee)
Sprained ankles
Hip pain

What would happen to a runner if they sprained their ankle and couldn't run for six weeks? Or damaged the ligaments in their knee and could never run again?

If running is all they enjoyed, they'd in all likelihood be devastated.

In this example we're using running, but this could be any sport or activity. Many people have one activity and one activity only that they truly enjoy.

This is where cross training comes into play. Using running as an example again, there's nothing wrong with loving to run! It's a great activity and millions of people enjoy it immensely. But when a person cross trains, they are actually helping themselves become better in their primary sport and increasing their overall conditioning. The key here is to find exercises that don't use the same muscles as used in the primary sport.

For example, runners shouldn't use walking, stair master, or similar exercises as a cross training exercise because they are, in essence, using the same muscles in a similar manner.

Not only that, they still aren't using muscles they don't use while running.

Good cross training exercises for runners would be things like swimming, weight training, and yoga.

With these exercises, they are getting a good workout while giving the primary muscles used in running a break.

Remember: This book is about being as physically, mentally and spiritually fit as you can be, and when applied to physical fitness, that means your entire body not just certain parts, inside and out.
When it comes to cross training, it all comes down to what YOU like, because if you enjoy it, you'll do it more often and with more enthusiasm.

On a personal note, I've had knee problems over the years, and if it weren't for cross training with the cycling, swimming, and weight training, I would've been forced to stop running years ago. My knees would be too damaged.

Thankfully, I found activities I enjoyed as much as running, so when I couldn't run, I was okay.

It's the same with you. Be creative and open minded! No one is saying you have to replace running or find something you enjoy just as much, but ask yourself: *"If I couldn't run (or pick your favorite sport) ever again, what would I do?"*

Try different activities and see how they feel!

Several years ago I was flipping channels and saw something I had never seen before:

It was two pro football players doing yoga. I couldn't believe what I was seeing. I literally dropped the remote and got comfortable. I had to see what was going on!

Later in the show, they talked about how the exercises really helped them stay injury free and even helped prolong their careers.

I was speechless.

I always thought yoga was for women. I thought guys didn't do yoga. We ran! We lifted weights! We hit stuff!

"Downward Dog is for women ONLY!!"

That was my opinion on yoga for years. Even decades.

But if these future Hall of Fame football players are doing it for the WORLD to see, then I need to check it out!

So now the question is, How do I go about trying it?

I was afraid to go to a class out of fear and embarrassment. I thought people would be staring at me or making fun of me. (I did not know anyone who looked like me who did yoga!) I thought I'd look silly trying to do the poses and I'd be shamed and made a spectacle.

To avoid all that, I decided to find yoga shows on television and record those. This way, I could try them in the privacy of my own home and could quit whenever I wanted.

I found a show and recorded a couple episodes. I'm nervous and excited at the same time! I'm thinking all types of stuff like, *What will happen? Will I like it?? What's all the excitement about? It looks so easy. This isn't even a workout!*

I finally play the recording. One of the very first moves we did was the Child's Pose. I get into the pose and within SECONDS I feel GREAT!

I couldn't believe the INSTANT PLEASURE I felt in my shoulders!

This is a pose where you are kneeling on your knees, face down, and arms extended forward. Being a swimmer, I had a little nagging pain in my right shoulder, but nothing major. This one simple move made me feel better almost instantly.

I was hooked. Within five minutes I knew I'd be doing yoga the rest of my life.

That was eight years ago and I still practice regularly.

Then there were other moves that I really enjoyed, especially the moves that helped stretch my back. Being on a bike for 2-4 hours at a time can be tough on your back, so these moves really helped loosen me up and brought my spine back into alignment.

Another benefit is how it affects me mentally. I noticed my mental state is slightly different for each activity I do. For example, running makes me feel one way, lifting weights makes me feel another way, while yoga makes me feel another way as well. They're entirely different exercises, but each of them have their physical and mental benefits.

This is one aspect that isn't discussed much. Personally, swimming takes more out of me than any other activity. I have to be really focused and mentally prepared to swim, as it really tires me out (mentally AND physically).

On the other hand, running doesn't take as much mental focus for me, while lifting weights does. When lifting heavy weights, it's important I pay attention to what I'm doing or risk injury. So, depending on how I'm feeling that day, I can elect to do any given training session and still get a good workout.

Ask yourself: What if one day you aren't mentally prepared to do your favorite activity? Do you not work out at all, or do something else?

That's another benefit of cross training.

When I tried yoga for the first time, I got angry at myself for being so closed minded and ignorant. I then realized how important it is to stay OPEN MINDED and not be so quick to dismiss exercises and activities.

Especially activities that have been around for thousands of years. Some of these yoga moves are very difficult and the toughest of tough guys would have trouble with them.

I also realized that there's a whole world out there I know NOTHING about, and if I'm not receptive to different ideas and challenges I could miss out on something that could help me.

I can honestly say that yoga has extended my swimming life. If my shoulder would've gotten worse, I would've been forced to cut back.

If I can't swim on a consistent basis, I can't do triathlons. No triathlons, and I probably wouldn't be a personal trainer. No personal trainer, no idea to write this book.

Funny how things work...

Am I saying that yoga is for everyone? Or a triathlon is the best cross training activity? No, not at all. What I'm saying is cross training in a variety of sports that work different muscles may lead you to discover different opportunities and activities you didn't know existed.

My favorite activity is lifting weights. Nothing beats pumping iron for me. But if the doctor told me I must stop lifting, I'd survive because I have other activities that I enjoy. I wouldn't be happy about not lifting, but I'd have other activities to enjoy. My workouts would continue and my fitness levels wouldn't take a tremendous hit.

How about you? If you couldn't do your favorite activity, what would you do?

If you're not sure, now's a great time to find out. Here are some great exercises and the calories a person can burn in 60 minutes. Expand your horizons and try something new. Your body will thank you!

Activity (one hour duration)	160 pounds (73 kilograms)	200 pounds (91 kilograms)	240 pounds (109 kilograms)
	Calories burned by bodyweight		
Aerobics, high impact	511	637	763
Aerobics, water	292	364	436
Basketball game	584	728	872
Bicycling < 10mph leisure	292	364	436
Bowling	219	273	327
Boxing	844	1110	1300
Dancing, ballroom	219	273	327
Diving, springboard, platform	211	245	279
Football, flag	584	728	872
Gardening, general	281	327	400
General housework	246	286	326
Golf, carrying clubs	329	410	491
Hiking	438	546	654
Ice Skating	511	637	763
Jogging 5mph	584	728	872
Mowing lawn, walking	387	449	512
Raquetball	511	637	763
Rollerblading	913	1138	1363
Rope jumping	730	910	1090
Rowing, stationary	511	637	763
Running, 8 mph	986	1229	1472
Skiing, cross country	511	637	763
Softball/baseball	365	455	545
Stair climbing, gym	657	819	981
Shoveling snow	422	490	558
Swimming, laps	511	637	763
Tae kwon do	730	910	1090
Tennis	584	728	872
Volleyball	292	364	436
Walking, 3.5 mph	277	346	414
Weightlifting, free weights	219	273	327

CHAPTER 8: AGING GRACEFULLY

As you can now see, there are many factors that can affect a person reaching their full physical potential. With all that said, there is one thing that's often conveniently overlooked: Our bodies change over time.

No matter how hard we try to prevent it or pretend it doesn't happen, we are getting older and our bodies are going through significant changes along the way.

Many of the changes are inevitable. We may be able to slow down some of these changes, but they WILL occur.

This is where "aging gracefully" comes into play.

It's important to know WHAT the changes are, because the latest exercise craze won't tell you about the changes. They will talk about the fantastic results you'll obtain, but those changes may not be realistic for everyone. It's also important to be MENTALLY prepared for these PHYSICAL challenges. (See how they tie in to each other?)

Not to mention, some of the exercises might be too dangerous for you.

The same goes for the diet plans. As we age, our nutritional needs might change also.

This knowledge is crucial for your mental fitness. There's nothing worse than going into a new training program or diet with the hopes of obtaining the body you had 10, 20, or 30 years ago.

You work hard and you don't see the progress you were expecting. Yes, there's some progress, but nothing like you were told to expect.

Many people go through this and give up out of frustration. They think the plans don't work and decide it's not worth the effort.

Sometimes a change in mindset is all that's needed to help a person see that they ARE making progress, and even though it's slow, it's steady progress.

When listening to a cell phone commercial or a new car commercial, the last 10 seconds are for the disclaimers and are said EXTREMELY fast.

The same type of disclaimer should be given for exercise and fitness.

Here are some facts:

1. Body fat increases with age.
The average person's body fat starts to increase after age 30.

2. Muscle loss.
After age 30, people tend to lose lean tissue. This process of muscle loss is called atrophy. Bones may lose some of their minerals and become less dense, making a person prone to osteoporosis. Tissue loss reduces the amount of water in your body.

3. Loss of height.
Height loss is related to aging changes in the bones, muscles, and joints. People typically lose about 1 cm (0.4 inches) every 10 years after age 40. Height loss is even more rapid after age 70. A person could lose a total of 1 to 3 inches in height as they age.

4. Weight gain (and loss).

Changes in total body weight vary for men and women. Men often gain weight until about age 55, and then begin to lose weight later in life. This may be related to a drop in the male sex hormone testosterone. Women usually gain weight until age 65, and then begin to lose weight.

5. Decreased mobility.

Less muscle in the legs and stiffer joints can make moving around harder. Excess body fat and changes in body shape also affect your balance, making falls more likely.

6. Changes in skin.

Skin can become less flexible, thinner, and more fragile. Skin can also bruise easily. Wrinkles, age spots, and skin tags may be more prominent. Decreased natural skin oil production can result in more dry and itchy skin.

There's nothing fun or exciting about reading these things. None of us want to envision these changes happening to us, but this is the raw reality. This is a normal part of the aging process.

This is just a small sample of the changes the body goes through. There are many medical publications that really get into detail about how our bodies change as we age, so we won't dwell on the changes themselves. The purpose here is to let you know these changes are NORMAL. Many of these changes you will experience at some point in your life.

The changes might be inevitable, but how extreme these changes are might be something you can control!

Not too long ago, I had some serious issues with getting older. Our society is geared toward younger people. As much as we'd like to deny it, age discrimination does exist. Then there was the thought that I wouldn't be able to do some of the things I could do when I was in my 20s. I saw many people older than me who have many physical ailments and are a shell of their former selves. They are in nursing homes, can't take care of themselves and are sickly.

Let's be honest: No one wants to live like that or looks forward to being in that condition.

While there are many seniors who fit that description, there are many that do NOT.

As I looked back over my life, I've had many positive, inspirational interactions with people 20, 30, even 40 years older than myself. In college, I had many professors who were in their 60s. My son's pediatrician is in his late 60s. In each case, they were youthful, energetic, and VERY mentally sharp.

But the biggest inspiration comes from the sport I love: Triathlon.

In football they have a saying: *"Look like Tarzan, play like Jane."* That basically means the guy *looks* very intimidating and like he can play very well, but in reality he's not very good.

He's terrible, actually.

It's the same with triathlon to an extent. You can't judge a book by its cover in this sport. There are some athletes who look extremely fit and fast, but aren't that good. On the flipside, a person who you think is slow as molasses may be one of the fastest people there.

When competing in a triathlon, you compete in age groups, ranging from 15-19, 24-29, 40-44, 65-69, etc. In some races, they also have divisions for those heavier than 200 pounds (which I'd race in). When you check in the morning of the race, all athletes get "marked." Your race number is written on your shoulder and your age is written on your calf. There's no hiding here. Everyone knows how old you are!

When I first got into the sport, I was pretty naive. I *ASS-U-MED* I was faster than every single competitor in their 40s and above. I was supremely confident and foolishly ignorant. How could anybody 20 years older than me be faster than me? Thirty years older than me? Please. Don't hurt yourself, old man! Aren't they *ALL* old and out of shape?

If you look at the primary sports (baseball, basketball, football, Olympic sports, etc.) most of the athletes are in their 20s and 30s. Most athletes competing in their late 30s and beyond are considered rare specimens. Most older people are out of shape and past their prime.

That's how I thought. Sad but true. Please excuse my ignorance, but surely I'm not the only one. Sometimes, a person needs to be shown live and in person how WRONG they are. A good butt kicking is in order!

So now, it's race day, 1995. I'm in Clermont, Florida to do a sprint triathlon: 400-yard swim, 11-mile bike, 3-mile run. This is my second triathlon and I'm EXCITED! My first race was just an introduction to the sport. I didn't know what I was doing, but I did enough to know I was HOOKED and couldn't wait to do another one!

Going into this race, my strategy was simple: pace myself on the swim and bike, then DESTROY the competition on the run. I came from a running background where I was running 6-7 minute miles. I was looking to place very well. Getting passed by ANYONE on the run was out of the question!

Even though I was a lifeguard in college, I wasn't the fastest swimmer. I don't enjoy getting kicked or swam over, so I like to start the swim towards the back, on the left side. Since my right side is my dominant side, I can swim and see everyone on my right when I breathe. This way, I don't have to worry about someone coming up behind me or from my left. It's a simple strategy that I still use to this day.

The swim starts and I'm swimming comfortably. Four hundred yards takes me about 7 minutes. You're still within striking distance of the leaders. The bike is another strategic portion for me. I ride the first 1/2 mile or so at a moderate pace to get my bearings, but after that, I HAMMER! Ride as hard as I can!

I pass a lot of people, but get passed also. I don't worry because the run is where it's won or lost, and the run is my ace in the hole! Another trick I learned is to ride an easier gear the last 1/2 mile or so to loosen your legs a bit for the run. Sometimes, your legs can feel like BRICKS when getting off the bike, and trying to run can be really tough, especially if you're running on sand.

So far, my plan is working to perfection. I glide into the transition area, rack my bike, put on my running shoes, and start running. I don't start out using my full stride, I run with a shorter, quicker turnover to loosen up my legs and prevent any leg cramps.

By mile 1 of the run I'm starting to feel pretty good! I'm not running my full stride, but I'm passing people who over did it on the bike. At mile 2, I'm cruising now. It wasn't my old 6-minute pace, but around 7-8 minutes. I'm really moving. I distinctly remember a guy saying, *"You run like an antelope!"* as I passed him. I replied, *"This antelope is tired!"* We both laughed, but I kept pushing my pace.

But then, it happens.

At mile 2.5 I'm really pushing hard. My motto is to *"Leave it on the field."* I don't want to look back on my race (or anything for that matter) and think I could've done more. I'm pushing as hard as I can.

Now mind you, I'm 27 years old at the time, at 6 feet tall, 170 pounds, and 4% body fat. Remember my feelings on people in their 40s, 50s and 60s? *Yeah, they're in shape, but I'll still smoke them!*

But all the sudden, this guy catches me. Then passes me. He has grey hair. I'm like, *Whoa! This dude is FLYING!* I look down at his calf where they put your age. I couldn't believe what I saw. This MUST be a misprint!

This man was 66 years old.

SIXTY SIX.

If THAT wasn't bad enough, he had the NERVE to say, *"Nice pace! Keep it up!"*

What??

In the sport of triathlon, people are VERY supportive and encouraging. It's a great atmosphere and everyone is welcome. If you cross the finish line, you're a winner! But when he passed me, I wanted to go crawl under a rock.

He passed me like I was standing still, and there was NOTHING I could do about it. In track and field, if someone passes you quickly, you get "walked." He passed me like I was WALKING. I was stunned. It was all fun and games when I passed that one guy, but things took a dramatic turn for the worst when I got passed by a guy old enough to be my father! How could this happen? Did he jump the course? There must be some explanation for this extraordinary event? No, he just beat me fair and square!

At that moment I knew I wasn't as good as I thought I was. It was a very humbling experience. As I did more triathlons, I saw so many older, fitter athletes that I didn't think twice about it. Especially the ones who do Ironman and half Ironman distances.

I distinctly remember racing in Ironman Florida 70.3 a couple years ago and I'm about 40 miles into the 56-mile bike portion.

I'm riding at a decent pace, nice and relaxed, when this older woman passes me.

She had grey hair, but that's all I could really see as she zipped past me.

Easily.

I glanced down at her calf and caught her age: 60. To make a long story short, somebody's GRANDMOTHER passed me like I was standing still. AGAIN. Unfortunately, I have more examples of people 20 and 30 years my senior faster than myself, but I think my point has been made.

Quite frankly, it's a tad embarrassing to be passed like that, and I'm glad there's no video of these events floating around. But on the flipside, I've passed people who were 10-20 years younger than myself, so I guess it's all relative!

The same way I talk about a 60-year-old is probably how a 20-something-year-old talks about me!

So I share my personal examples of shame and humiliation because many feel that getting older is a death sentence, but it doesn't have to be. We can't stop the aging process, but we can slow it down with diet, exercise, and living a positive, stress-free lifestyle.

Instead of dreading the aging process, accept it for what it is. If you don't want to get old, the only other alternative is death. Accept the fact you're getting older and look at it as a challenge. It took me seeing phenomenal athletes 20-30 years my senior to inspire me to push myself.

There was a time when I was embarrassed to tell people how old I was. I associated getting older with negative connotations. I would watch events on television like the NFL Combine, where the top college players in the country would participate in various drills for the pro scouts and coaches and I'd get frustrated that I wasn't on their level physically.

What I had to accept (which was hard to do at times) was the fact that not only are they elite athletes, but they are at least 20 years YOUNGER than me. Comparing myself to them was a waste of my time, and when I did, my wife would quickly say *"well, you're no spring chicken!"* She was right, but who cares? I wasn't trying to hear that!

Getting upset or sad wasn't helping me be the best I could be. I had to make a choice: either change my mindset or be miserable and feel sorry for myself.

I decided to choose the former.

I refuse to use my getting older as an excuse to "let myself go." On the contrary, I look at getting older as a challenge and an opportunity to see how good of shape I can get in. People can tell you something, but it's much more convincing when you see it for yourself, and seeing older people excel in sports is inspiring.

So, I say lead by example. Use the fact that you're getting older to motivate others to take care of themselves. Show them the way. Take care of yourself so your quality of life stays good as you age. In addition to using those who are in great shape as motivation, use those who are NOT in the best of health as motivation also.

Don't use your age as an excuse to not try or excel. This is an important aspect of being mentally fit. Tell yourself you will succeed *"in spite of."*

Using triathlon as another example, the Ironman is considered the ultimate in endurance events, with the world championship in Hawaii as being the #1 goal for triathletes around the world. The 2.4 mile swim, 112 mile bike and 26.2 mile run requires you to be in peak physical condition. There's no handicap division or breaks. Either finish in 17 hours, or your time doesn't count. Everyone is equal.

Most people can't do either of the three disciplines by themselves, let alone all three in the same day; but, Lew Hollander and Harriet Anderson can. The fact that a person can finish at all is amazing, but what makes this even more astounding is Lew is 82 years old and Harriet is 78! They are the oldest Ironman finishers at the time I wrote this.

Think about that for a minute. An 82-year-old and 78-year-old completing a 2.4 mile swim, 112 mile bike, and a full marathon! In the same day? Society would tell you it's impossible, but it has been done. Don't let your age dictate what you can or can't do. The instant you start to tell yourself you can't do something is the day you stop living. I wonder how many people told Lew Hollander that doing Ironman at his age is crazy and extremely dangerous. How many people have the courage to climb Mount Everest at ANY age, let alone the age of 80 like Yuichiro Miura? How many people may have tried to tell him to find something less strenuous?

I'm not suggesting you go out and do Ironman or try to climb Mount Everest. These are extreme examples, but they also show that you can't use your age as an excuse to not get out there and live life to the fullest. If taken care of, the human body is capable of performing at a high level for decades.

Our society tells us to retire at age 65. Take it easy and "enjoy your 'Golden Years.'

A person may be retired from work, but they're not retired from life.

Don't let society or anyone you know prevent you from living your life to the fullest, no matter how old you are. There's no age limit to being the best person you can be. The philosophies in this book are the blueprint to aging gracefully. It's even more important that you're taking care of yourself as you age, and that includes the following tips:

Diet

As we age, it's critical that we watch what we eat. Foods we ate as a teen or young adult may be difficult for us to digest as we get older. Not only that, it's important we keep our immune system as strong as we can to help fend off age related illnesses such as cancer, arthritis, macular degeneration, Alzheimer's, brittle bones, etc.

The foods we eat can go a long way in helping us age gracefully. The key to aging gracefully is to start eating these foods on a consistent basis NOW, not when you hit 40 or 50.

Brittle bones

As we age, our bones tend to get weaker and more brittle. Here are foods that can help keep the bones strong:

Kale
Cottage cheese
Cabbage
Collard greens
Yogurt
Fortified milk
Cheese
Sardines
Salmon
Spinach
Fortified cereals

Mental health

Many people tend to become forgetful or can't seem to stay focused as they age. Here are some great foods for mental fitness:

Fish
Whole grains (oatmeal, brown rice, barley)
Beans
Eggs
Turkey
Leafy greens (spinach, romaine lettuce, turnip, and mustard greens)

Broccoli
Yogurt
Almonds

Dental health

Once we lose our baby teeth, that's it! In addition to daily brushing and flossing, eat these foods to keep your teeth strong, cavity free, and to minimize stains:

Raisins
Water
Broccoli
Carrots
Apples
Cucumbers
Cranberries
Almonds

Digestion

Bloating, acidity, abdominal discomfort, and nausea are problems people of all ages deal with, but can be especially hard on an older person. Keep your digestive system strong and working efficiently with these foods:

Tomatoes
Beets
Ginger
Carrots
Cantaloupe
Apples
Peaches
Bananas
Lemon water
Sweet potatoes
Avocados
Oatmeal
Blueberries

Eyesight

Our vision tends to diminish as we age, but these foods can help keep your eyes healthy. There is no known way to totally stop the decrease in vision, but it's still suggested that these foods be eaten on a regular basis:

Kale
Spinach
Peanut butter
Tuna
Mackerel
Oranges
Peas
Broccoli
Milk
Shellfish
Carrots
Romaine lettuce
Grapefruit juice
Cauliflower
Sunflower seeds
Almonds
Oysters

Healthy skin

Our skin takes a beating over the years with acne, scrapes, bumps and bruises, etc. Then of course there's sunburn and the long term effects of over exposure to the sun. In addition to using sunscreen and general skin care maintenance, eat these foods to keep your skin healthy from the inside out:

Sunflower seeds
Pomegranate
Yogurt
Walnuts
Peppers
Dark chocolate
Kidney beans

Soy
Oatmeal
Green tea

Healthy heart

This is the one muscle that we MUST keep working if we want to age gracefully! Eat these foods to keep your heart strong, as well as to decrease your risk of heart disease and minimize any circulation issues:

Oatmeal
Blueberries
Nuts (almonds, walnuts, pecans, peanuts, etc.)
Salmon
Tofu
Tuna
Brown rice
Red wine
Onions
Oranges
Squash
Green tea
Cantaloupe
Papaya
Sweet potatoes
Asparagus
Carrots
Broccoli
Garlic
Watermelon
Pineapples
Olive oil

There are many, many books that go into more detail about diet and the best foods to eat. The goal here is to give you a general idea as to what types of foods a person should eat to age gracefully.

This list is incomplete, as there are MANY other foods a person can eat that will help them. Grapefruit, raspberries, grapes, green beans, squash, etc. are just a few foods not mentioned above that have fantastic health benefits.

There is no one magical food. The key is to eat a variety of foods to ensure you're getting the nutrients your body needs.

However, at the same time, notice the foods NOT on the list of suggested foods:

Cakes
Cookies
Potato chips
Soda
Fast food
Alcoholic beverages

Many of these products are harmful to your body and will actually age you. Sugar, processed meats, excess sodium and fried foods should be eaten sparingly if at all. I must be honest: I still eat some of the foods that are considered bad for you.

I'm a firm believer in "cheat days," where you can eat what you enjoy. The key is to not have cheat days every day! An occasional treat every now and then should not hurt you (once a week for me), but at the same time, if you have any medical issues, consult with your doctor about what you can and can't eat.

Don't get to the point where your doctor forbids you from eating something. Once you get to that point you're in a dangerous place health wise. Not only that, it means you've been indulging in your bad foods for a very long time, and now you have to quit cold turkey. Quitting ANYTHING cold turkey is very difficult, and is even harder when you are being forced to.

DO NOT GET TO THIS POINT, AS YOU WILL BE MISERABLE! If you know something you eat isn't good for you, start cutting back on it NOW and start taking better care of yourself TODAY. It may be difficult but in time you'll be glad you did, because eventually you can eat your favorite food sparingly and guilt free.

There are people out there who never eat junk or fast food. That's perfectly fine. Maybe even ideal, but I still enjoy those foods. I'm a firm believer in moderation. Life is too short to be serious and strict ALL THE TIME.

Another benefit of eating healthy is you will start to feel better. Many people are afraid to get older because they fear many of the age related illnesses that they see people endure. Eating many of the healthy foods listed above helps keep your immune system strong, and a strong immune system is the first line of defense against illness and disease.

The key here is to be proactive, and take care of your body NOW, and to not rely on a doctor to prescribe expensive medication that may or may not make you better. That's the key to aging gracefully. Change your diet and you change your life!

I can guarantee you that Lew Hollander is enjoying his life. Same for Harriet Anderson and Yuichiro Miura. If they can enjoy their life and age gracefully, why can't you? What's stopping YOU from living your life to the fullest?

CHAPTER 9: BODY IMAGE & THE MEDIA

At this point, you can see that there's more to being physically fit than just working out. Nutrition, age, and rest play a significant part. Knowing your body type (ectomorph, endomorph or mesomorph) is an important part of becoming the best you can be physically, as well as helping you keep your goals (and results) realistic.

In addition to the physical aspect of working out, the mental aspect is just as important. It's imperative that people remember that and work on their mental fitness as they work on their physical fitness.

In other words, it's important to be comfortable with who you are and accept the body type you are given. If you're not comfortable in your own skin, have self-hatred or a negative body image, it's practically impossible to be the best you can be.

We ALL have flaws. We ALL have a certain body part or feature we don't like about ourselves. Personally, I have sensitive skin and I'm prone to breakouts. But instead of dwelling on my imperfections, I work to make them better, while at the same time accepting them and not beating myself up for not being "perfect," or being envious of someone who I feel has better skin than I do.

I am at peace with my flaws. Am I still working to improve them? Absolutely. But at the same time, I'm not going to let them stop me from reaching my full potential! For some, this is hard to do for a variety of reasons. But one very important reason people have a hard time is because they are bombarded with images of beauty or perfection every day. When a person turns on the television, opens a magazine or looks at an advertisement, they may not see someone who looks like them.

Matter of fact, they may see someone who looks NOTHING like them, so they may feel left out or excluded. Or, on the flip-side, the person who DOES look like them is portrayed in a negative light. The person who looks like them is the nerd or the ugly, unpopular one.

The lack of diverse images in the media can have a tremendous effect on a person's self-esteem, how they see themselves, and how OTHERS view them as well. How difficult is it to be motivated to look your best by exercising and living a healthy lifestyle when those you see in the public eye don't look like you or aren't considered attractive?

How difficult is it to work out as an endomorph when you want to look like an mesomorph, because that's all you see on television or in the magazines? This is an aspect of exercise and fitness that a person must be aware of, because it may be subliminally holding them back.

There have been numerous studies that have shown us how the media can lead to a negative perception of a person's body image. The movie and music industries, as well as advertisements, constantly portray an ideal and beautiful body for women that has changed over the years.

When people see these images and then look at their own bodies, which are often times different from what is portrayed as ideal in the media, they begin to think that they aren't beautiful, are too fat, too pale, etc. This dissatisfaction with one's body image can lead to low self-esteem, and even depression.

It's very difficult to be the best person you can be if you base your beauty on what you see in the media, as it is constantly changing. For example, let's look at the ideal standards of beauty for women over the past several decades:

The 1940s and early 1950s marked voluptuous and curvaceous sweater girls, also known as "pin-up" girls, e.g. Sophia Loren and Marilyn Monroe (the quintessential American sex symbol).

British teen model Twiggy came on the scene in the 1960s when slenderness became the most significant indicator of physical attractiveness.

In the 1970s there was a continued emphasis on weight loss and body shape. The media used thinner, less curvaceous models in photo shoots. Charlie's Angel star Farrah Fawcett had one of the most sought-after body types.

The 1980s beauty ideal remained slim but required a more toned and fit look. This decade was known as the age of the supermodel, e.g. Cindy Crawford and Naomi Campbell. Dieting was no longer enough to fit into the correct size; there was now the added pressure of exercise (aerobics craze) to achieve the toned look.

The 1990s ideal body was very skinny and large breasted, i.e. Pamela 'Baywatch' Anderson. This was called the "Barbie look." At the same time, thinness was continuing to stay strong as model Kate Moss was extremely popular in Calvin Klein advertisements.

More recently, in the 2000s, the ideal shape is one that may have to be purchased and cultivated through artificial means (plastic surgery, liposuction, breast and butt enhancements, etc.).

In essence, women are buying (and chasing) an unattainable fantasy.

Now keep in mind, there are three basic body types. There's a very good chance your body type is NOT in "style" at the present time. If that's the case, that does NOT make you less attractive than what the media portrays as attractive.

Just because your body type is not on the cover of your favorite magazine doesn't mean you shouldn't work hard to be the best person you can be. It's important to remember that beauty comes in all shapes and sizes.

You must be mentally strong and know that true beauty comes from WITHIN, not from a magazine editor's opinion.

Unfortunately, a lot of people follow what the media says is attractive. They are looking to the media to define what the ideal standard of beauty is, but as you can see, it has changed over the decades.

This will particularly affect younger people, as they want to fit in and be accepted.

In a perfect world, we'd see all ages, races, creeds and colors portrayed positively in the media. Unfortunately, that's not the case. Many segments of the population are either not represented or shown in a negative light the majority of the time.

There is beauty in ALL shapes, sizes, and colors, but it's not shown as much as it should be.

The media has its own agenda. Their primary goal is to make money, not to be morally responsible to the masses.

If a certain look or image will make money, that image will be what you see.

It's even more imperative we stop relying on the media for the standards of beauty because we are living in a technologically advanced age. Our televisions, computers, cell phones, even our cars are extremely tech savvy. These advances have made many of our lives easier, but there's one aspect in which it has made it worse for quite a few of us.

PHOTOSHOPPING

Not to be confused with Adobe Photoshop, the program developed and published by Adobe Systems, "photoshopping" is the practice of altering photos of people, in many cases for magazines and photos posted online. This is done primarily to make people look "better," and is widely used by mainstream media for magazine covers. The cover is what gets people's attention, thus prompting them to buy the magazine. The more people buy the magazine, the more advertisers can be charged to solicit their goods in that magazine. The more they charge, the greater their profits. The greater the profits, the happier the shareholders.

Photoshopping is not just fun and games; it's big business. Photoshop was created in 1988 by Thomas and John Knoll. Since then, it has become the "de facto" industry standard in raster graphics editing. There are many other companies that now offer image editing tools and software similar to Adobe Photoshop, but many will use the generic term "photoshopped" no matter what company's software they are using.

Please note: Adobe Photoshop and the other similar programs do much more than make people look thin. (My book cover was created using imaging software.) Using these software tools to alter human's bodies is the problem, not the companies who created them.

It may be lucrative, but there's a lot of controversy about using digitally enhanced photos, because many say it's seriously affecting an entire generation's body image and making people feel worse about themselves and their appearance.

So how big an issue is modifying photos in advertising?

According to a retoucher who spoke on a condition of anonymity, it's very widespread:

"There's just no way an image would be released without any retouching at all so every single ad would have that disclaimer on it. And absolutely 100 percent of what's in fashion magazines is retouched... You can never have no retouching across the board, because some of it you just have to do if something's really distracting in a picture."

They went on to say:

"We completely remove veins and freckles and moles and bags under the eyes all the time. We often remove body hair, subdue wrinkles, whiten teeth, pop the eyes. We also smooth kneecaps and veins in the hands and things like that — anything that's distracting that takes away from the product being featured."

Then there's the practice of "Frankensteining."

"But retouchers do things like cut out a head from one photo and put it on the body from another. I do that kind of stuff all the time. Let's say they do a photo-shoot with a model and the body comes out well, but she's got a wonky look on her face. They might want to put this head on that body. Or they want to put an arm from one photo on the body of another — that's common."

This is VERY important for many different reasons. When people see these images which, in essence, are perfect, they then look at themselves and see someone who doesn't look as good. So now, you have a person who's working out and exercising diligently to look like their favorite celebrity or athlete, but the look they're trying to attain was retouched and/or photoshopped.

What they may not realize is the pictures have been altered. The very things they find pleasing in the picture don't exist. They're trying to look like something that isn't even real.

According to many studies, this "normal" practice is very damaging to a young girl's self-esteem.

According to recent studies, nearly 50% of girls under the age of six are worried that they're fat, and by the age of 17, 78% of girls say they are unhappy with their bodies. Certainly, low self-esteem is a problem, but there are long-term psychological and medical issues to consider as well. According to the National Association of Anorexia Nervosa and Associated Disorders, as many as 10 million women in America suffer from some form of eating disorder.

The statistics are alarming, so much so that the American Medical Association has taken notice. In 2011, the AMA adopted a new policy to "encourage advertising associations to work with public and private sector organizations to establish guidelines that would discourage airbrushing or retouching in advertising, especially those appearing in teen-oriented publications."

Barbara McAneny, an AMA board of trustee's physician, told the press, *"[We've] had enough. We must stop exposing impressionable children and teenagers to advertisements portraying models with body types only attainable with the help of photo editing software."*

Altering images has become such a large problem that in other countries, the political world is taking notice. Indeed, legislation was introduced in 2009 in France that would require retouched ads to carry a label disclosing that fact; similar proposals are circulating in the United Kingdom and Norway.

Not only women are affected by this issue; men are as well. Men are visual creatures. A woman's physical attractiveness is an important factor for who many will date and are attracted to. As young girls are affected by enhanced images , young boys are too. They see these photoshopped images and think that is what women are supposed to look like.

As girls are hard on themselves to look a certain way, boys tease girls who don't look a certain way also. This is unhealthy for all involved. They don't understand that the image they are seeing isn't real. It's just an illusion.

But it's not just women who are being photoshopped. The photoshopping of men has been steadily on the rise over the years.

Their vision of beauty is just as distorted as that of a young girl's, and it appears as though the pressure on men to look fit and have unrealistic bodies is higher than ever. According to the BBC, men are facing similar pressures as women to look good and it is contributing to a rise in the numbers having cosmetic surgery, experts say.

The Men's Health Forum said advertising and the media were reinforcing the stereotypes that men needed to be athletic-looking and toned. The number of men over 50 having cosmetic surgery has risen more than 140% in five years.

Liposuction comes out on top as the favorite procedure. One in four of all liposuction operations carried out by The Harley Medical Group are now on men, the firm said. Peter Baker, chief executive of the Men's Health Forum, said:

"Many men need to eat more healthily and do more exercise. But the rise is also to do with the increasing pressures men now face. Since the late 80s and early 90s, the message to men is that they have to look good. We constantly see images of men with six-packs and toned bodies on the front of magazines and on TV. It is similar to what women have had to put up with for much longer, although it is not yet as bad. It is unhelpful."

Pro tennis star Andy Roddick appeared on a popular magazine cover and was surprised at the end result:

Roddick is quoted as saying*: "I'm not as fit as the Men's Fitness cover suggests...little did I know I have 22 inch guns and a disappearing birth mark on my right arm... I walked by the newsstand in the airport and did a total double take...it was pretty funny...whoever did this has mad skills."*

As you can see, the practice of altering images is firmly entrenched in our society and it doesn't appear to be slowing down any time soon. Many fitness and weight loss products use image editing software as well to prompt people eager to lose weight and get in shape to purchase those products.

It's very important to acknowledge that photoshopping exists and that many of the images you see are altered. Parents must talk to their daughters at an early age and let them know they are beautiful the way they are and that it's important to love themselves and be comfortable in their own skin.

Our sons need to be educated as well. What they see in the magazines is not reality, and they need to not compare girls to what they see in the magazines because they are in the business of selling fantasy. Society has put too much emphasis on trying to be "perfect." It's important for us ALL to remember we have flaws and to learn to love and accept ourselves.

As discussed before, there are different body types, and it's important you learn to love and accept yourself as you are. The premise of this book is to be the best you can be, and that includes mentally accepting your physical gifts, limitations and flaws. Constantly comparing yourself to others or feeling physically inadequate can hold you back in other aspects of your life.

Focus on being the best YOU can be, not what society says you should be. If history repeats itself, a new look will be popular a couple years from now and people will be trying to attain THAT look instead of working on their best, unique self.

It's time to stop this ridiculous cycle.

CHAPTER 10: THE DANGERS OF ADDICTION: PRESCRIPTION DRUGS

Here's one aspect of physical fitness that many overlook. Most of us know how bad illegal drugs are and how damaging they can be, but LEGAL drugs (prescription and over the counter, "OTC") can be just as bad, if not worse. People may feel that "just" taking medicine they buy at the local drugstore or taking medicine prescribed by their doctor is safe, but these have their dangers as well.

Accidental deaths involving medications are most often *not* from the medications themselves, but from an unapproved combination of medications and/or alcohol. Alcohol mixed with any medication can have negative side effects. However, the most dangerous medications mixed with alcohol include sleeping aids, anti-anxiety drugs, antihistamines, and anti-depressants.

When taking medicines, whether doctor prescribed or OTC, it's crucial that you know what you're taking, and to be wary when adding another medicine to your daily intake. *Always* let your doctor or pharmacist know what medicines you're taking, and ask him or her first before taking anything new.

It's also important to remember that drugs can linger in your body for days (or in some cases weeks) at a time. This is important when using a new medication. A person may not think they are mixing medicines because they don't take them on the same day, when in essence they are still mixing drugs because the other drug is still in their system from several days ago.

It's impossible to be at your physical, mental or spiritual best if you are addicted to drugs of ANY type.

Here is an approximate detection times chart for various drugs.

Drug	Minimum Drug Detection Time	Maximum Drug Detection Time
Amphetamines	2-7 hours	2-4 days
Barbiturates	2-4 hours	1-3 weeks
Benzodiazepines	2-7 hours	1-4 days
Cocaine	1-4 hours	2-4 days
Ecstasy	2-7 hours	2-4 days
Marijuana	2 hours	Up to 40 + days
Methamphetamine	2-7 hours	2-4 days
Methadone	3-8 hours	1-3 days
Opiates	2 hours	2-3 days
Oxycodone	1-3 hours	1-2 days
Tricyclic Antidepressants	8-12 hours	2-7 days

These are approximate detection times for the drug or metabolites in urine per the Mayo Clinic. The actual detection time depends on dose, frequency of use, and individual metabolism.

In its simplest terms, pain killers are nothing but mood altering drugs. When part of your body is injured, special nerve endings send pain messages back to your brain. Painkilling drugs interfere with these messages, either at the site of the injury, in the spinal cord or in the brain itself. Many drugs work by copying or blocking the effects of naturally occurring chemicals in your brain.

When cells in your body are injured or damaged, they release a chemical called prostaglandin.

When you take a pain reliever like ibuprofen, it keeps injured or damaged cells from making and releasing prostaglandin. When the cells don't release this chemical, it means that the brain won't get the pain message as quickly or clearly. So your pain goes away or becomes less severe for as long as the cells aren't releasing the chemical. Acetaminophen works in the brain so you don't feel the pain.

There's nothing wrong with taking a painkiller every now and then. The problem arises when a person keeps taking it for an extended period of time:

- The body generates less amounts of prostaglandin, because it is receiving it from an external source;
- The brain starts to increase the number of receptors for the drug;
- The body starts to become dependent on the external source of painkillers, and as a result, if a person attempts to stop, the body starts to go through withdrawals.

If a person continues to take it now to just avoid the withdrawal symptoms, they have become addicted. Taking painkillers for an extended period of time causes a change in one's brain chemistry that is not under the individual's control. Addiction is a chemical and physical disease, one that requires expert medical treatment in a safe, humane environment.

This is a simplified breakdown of drugs and how they affect your brain and how a person can become addicted.

Overdosing on OTC or prescription drugs can be deadly. Here's a brief list of celebrities who have died from prescription drugs, many of which you can get from a doctor's prescription or over the counter at the local drugstore:

Gerald Levert, 11-10-2006
Six drugs: including painkillers Vicodin, Percocet and Dextropropoxyphene (AKA Darvocet), sedative/anxiety medication alprazolam (AKA Xanax) and two non-prescription antihistamines

Anna Nicole Smith, 2-8-2007
Eleven drugs: including chloral hydrate (sleep aid) and several sedatives/muscle relaxants, clonazepam (AKA Klonopin), lorazepam (AKA Ativan), oxazepam (AKA Serax) and diazepam (AKA Valium)

Dorothy Dandridge, 9-8-1965
One drug: Imipramine, AKA Tofranil (antidepressant)

Heath Ledger, 2-6-2008
Six drugs: painkillers oxycodone and hydrocodone, sleep aid temazepam and sedatives diazepam (AKA Valium), alprazolam (AKA Xanax) and doxylamine

Pimp C, 12-4-2007
Two drugs: Promethazine (antihistamine) and codeine (painkiller)

Dana Plato, 5-8-1999
Two drugs: Carisoprodol, AKA Soma (muscle relaxant), and Vicodin (painkiller)

Michael Jackson, 6-25-2009
One drug: Propofol intoxication

Addiction is both a physical and mental problem, so this topic will be revisited in the Mental Fitness Section.

As you can see, there are many factors that must be taken into account when trying to become physically fit. Some of these may be affecting you on a subliminal level that you are unaware of, but not anymore! It's time. It's time to take full control of our lives. It's time to encompass ALL aspects of physical fitness so we can become the best we can be!

So far, we have looked at the individual and how they can help themselves, but many of us have loved ones who we have to factor into our quest for improved physical fitness. It's time to examine how we incorporate our loved ones into our lifestyle changes!

CHAPTER 11: IS MY MATE MAKING ME FAT?

One of the most exciting times in a person's life is meeting that special someone. You can't wait to see that person, and the mere THOUGHT of them makes your heart beat a little faster!

Early in the relationship, it's the "get to know you" phase. You're trying to spend as much time together as possible, doing as many fun things you can with each other.

For the guys, it's about trying to woo and impress. We want to show her a good time, and that includes taking her out and showing how much fun we are.

Many times that means doing things you don't normally do, such as going out to eat more often or spending a little more time with that person eating while cuddled up watching TV.

Both sides are enjoying each other's company and there's nothing wrong with that, but the concern is that you may not be as active as you used to be as a result.

According to an article in The Daily Mail UK, relationships are the number one cause for weight gain in Britain, ahead of comfort eating and indulging on a holiday.

The study conducted by Diet Chef shows that 62% of people gained weight after commencing a new relationship and another two-thirds of the people surveyed admitted to putting on weight together.

The survey has found that 52% of women eat as much as their male partner.

The survey also showed that relationship weight gain happens because couples have a tendency to nest in the early stages of their relationship. This means numerous nights relaxing with each other indoors.

As time goes on and the relationship progresses, we tend to spend more and more time with our partners and a little less time taking care of ourselves.

In actuality, there are many reasons for the weight gain in a relationship: pregnancy, kids, the gradual increase in weight as the years go by, lack of time to exercise, work and home responsibilities, etc.

These are all legitimate reasons and In upcoming sections we'll go over ways a couple or family can lose weight and become healthier together.

But there's one aspect of the weight gain that should be looked at from a mental fitness/personal growth perspective.

For some, the purpose of exercise and fitness is to make themselves attractive to suitable mates. They want to look good when they meet that special someone. At the same time, they may also believe the physical aspect of the relationship is *not* as important once they are in a long term relationship (i.e. marriage).

So as the months and years go by, a person may get comfortable and feel that their partner isn't going anywhere. They did all the hard work already by wooing that person and now they are in a committed relationship. As a result, they don't have to work as hard to stay in shape or keep up their physical appearance.

As a person gets more and more comfortable, their thought process starts to change:

"I got him. I don't have to work as hard now."

"She loves me for me, not because of how I look. If I gain a little weight, it's no big deal."

"It's not about 'us' anymore. It's about raising these kids. I don't have time to work out!"

"I'm married now. I just go to work and come home. What else is there?"

Not everyone feels this way (of course), but these thoughts and similar ones are quite common.

Now it very well could be true that their partner isn't going anywhere. Many people still believe in "till death do us part," but getting too comfortable isn't good for a person's health and fitness levels, as discussed in this book.

Being "comfortable" can prevent a person from becoming the best they can be in many aspects of their life.

I'd be leery of going to a doctor who felt so comfortable that he wasn't trying to learn about new medicines and remedies to treat his clients.

"Doc? What are these leeches for?"

Or the lawyer who passed the bar exam 15 years ago and didn't want to learn about new laws and court rulings that could impact his clients. He figured he passed the bar so his job was done.

How long would a pro basketball player last in the NBA if he stopped training after signing his contract?

We can think of many instances where getting too comfortable isn't a good thing, yet when it comes to relationships it's not only acceptable, it's thought to be a natural progression in a relationship.

I believe this is NOT acceptable.

Just because you're in a relationship doesn't mean you stop growing and evolving as a person. It's just the opposite: You now have a person you can grow with. You two can grow TOGETHER.

Many couples get into a rut or routine where they eventually start going through the motions. This could eventually stunt their growth and prevent them from living their lives to the fullest.

Whether you're in a relationship or not, life is meant to be lived and enjoyed, not just surviving one day to the next.

But for some, "settling down" means just that. They are settled. They have gotten all the partying and having a good time out of their system and are now ready to get with that one special person and live "happily ever after."

But in many cases, that includes getting into a mundane routine, gaining weight, boredom, becoming more sedentary and having an increased risk of health issues due to the weight gain.

This scenario is NOT part of being the best you can be physically, mentally and spiritually.

Some have not only settled, they've *stopped.* They've stopped living!

Yes, it's true you're in a relationship, but you're still your own person. Relationships do not mean you can't do some of the things you enjoyed while you were single. It's crucial you (and your mate) keep some of your individuality and continue to do some of the things you enjoyed, while growing and cultivating your relationship *at the same time.*

There's no law saying just because you're in a relationship that you MUST spend all your free time together. Sometimes you need a little space, even in the most perfect of relationships. Personally, I was doing triathlons years before I met my wife. I was also going out to clubs and having a good time as well. After we became exclusive, I stopped going out to clubs and spent that time with her instead. But at the same time, I continued to do triathlons.

I gave up something I enjoyed (clubbing), but at the same time, I was still able to do something I enjoyed very much (triathlons). My then girlfriend (and now wife) understood how important triathlons were to me and had no problem with my training, provided it didn't interfere with our time together.

In some instances, a person will try to change their partner by forcing them to do things HE likes to do, or preventing her from doing what SHE likes to do. Or she'll make him feel guilty for wanting to do things she disapproves of or doesn't like. All relationships require sacrifice and hard work, but that doesn't mean a person should sacrifice their happiness or ALL their independence for the sake of the relationship.

The growth in a relationship should be voluntary and mutually enjoyable for BOTH parties, not just for one.

It's important that both partners have a mutual respect for each other and be on the same page as far as what they want in the relationship and where it's headed.

Constantly trying to control your mate or making them feel guilty about things they enjoy could prompt them to resent you and not want to do anything but sit at home and be miserable. This lack of interest and unhappiness could lead to a variety of issues, including stress eating, which could lead to weight gain.

Even if you don't understand WHY your partner enjoys something, leaving them alone and letting them be may be the best thing for both of you.

As a health and fitness enthusiast, I'd give my wife advice and tips on exercises. She did NOT want my (unsolicited!) advice and had no intention of doing triathlons. She was perfectly content walking on the treadmill as she watched her soap operas!

It took me quite some time to come to the realization that she was HAPPY on her treadmill and that was her time to catch up on her soaps. It slowly dawned on me to just let her be. If that makes her happy, why try change it? Just because I like something doesn't mean she MUST like it also or should feel the same way about it as I do. She had a life before me. There's nothing wrong with doing some of the things she did before she met me.

I have since learned to leave her be on some things, and she has done the same with me. She thinks I'm CRAZY for wanting to ride my bike for four hours, or get up at 5:30 to train, but she doesn't try to stop me. She doesn't understand it, nor does she try to!

These simple gestures have allowed us to keep our individuality and not feel smothered in the relationship. We also eliminated the stress of thinking we are REQUIRED to like everything the other likes or be upset that they don't feel the same way.

We are keeping our individuality to a degree, but still growing together at the same time. If both partners are active and on the same page, that can help them stay mentally fit, as well as eliminating the stress of trying to make things work by force.

So will giving each other a little space and keeping a portion of their individuality prevent a person from gaining weight? Of course not, but it COULD help keep them refreshed and mentally fit by providing an outlet to eliminate some of the stress in their lives.

Remember: Being fit has several components and they work best when in unison.

A couple could be stress free and mentally refreshed as described above, but they are happily gaining weight together by eating unhealthy foods while watching TV. But that means they are not being physically fit. They're fine mentally, but lacking physically.

To be the best they can be (both together and as individuals), they should work on all aspects of their fitness together, as a team. Once they are on the same page and have their goals established, they can give each other support and encouragement when times get tough.

A strong support system is a wonderful thing to have, and if your mate is your biggest supporter and motivator that will make it that much easier for you to succeed.

On the flip-side, it's important to offer your partner as much support and encouragement as they give you. The idea is to help each other, and in doing so your bond will increase as you both reach your individual goals and the goals you set together as a team.

Being the best you can be physically, mentally and spiritually is great, but it can be that much better if your partner is on the same journey with you. This is where communication is key. Talk to your partner. Let them know what your goals are and WHY you have decided to make these changes.

Stress how important these goals are to you, and also how important it would be for them to go along with you on this journey. Let them know how it will benefit them as well.

Once you two are on the same page, nothing will stop you from achieving your goals!

CHAPTER 12: FAMILY FITNESS

The family fitness section encompasses all three aspects of fitness. Even though it's included in the physical fitness section, there are aspects that can apply to mental and spiritual fitness as well. We are slowly putting the pieces together!

Being fit is a personal endeavor. No one can make you fit. A person may have a coach, peers or other sources of motivation to push them, but at the end of the day, it's up to that individual to work as hard as they can to be the best they can be.

Personally, I think we all need to not only strive to be the best we can, but to be a source of inspiration to others.

There are many ways to inspire someone, as I discovered years ago. A good friend of mine said she became a personal trainer after I made a training program for her. She said she enjoyed it so much, she decided she wanted to become a personal trainer also.

Another person who I never met in person contacted me online and said my training blog inspired her to start swimming. Another said they looked forward to my daily motivational messages on my website (www.jeffwhitefitnesssolutions.com) and that it inspired them to never give up. I have received countless comments over the years from people I never met all over the world thanks to the Internet, and it's always much appreciated and inspires ME to keep going, even when I want to stop sometimes.

I bring that up to say this: You don't have to preach to someone or even know them to inspire them.

I have discovered "by accident" that people are always watching and observing others. I honestly had NO IDEA if people were reading my blogs, watching my fitness videos or anything—not until someone told me they were. So there are people watching YOU, RIGHT NOW. You are an inspiration as you read this and don't even realize it.

It could be anyone, anywhere:

A coworker at work who admires your work ethic; a classmate who marvels at your intelligence; or a person at the gym who sees you minding your own business, self-motivated and training hard.

Many times, you don't know they are watching. Personally, I use others for inspiration all the time, and many times they don't even know it. Surely I'm not the only one!

So with that being said, it shouldn't be hard to believe you're inspiring those close to you also. Even though I received inspiration from everyone—from peers and teachers to complete strangers—my biggest inspirations came from my family, especially my mother and uncles.

It wasn't necessarily what they said that inspired me, it's what they did, day in and day out. My uncles taught me work ethic and how a man should take care of his kids. They weren't absentee dads or abandoned their kids. They were there every day, doing the little things. As a kid, growing up without a father, I noticed that. I never said anything, but I noticed.

People will say, *"Do what I say, not what I do."* We've all heard something similar, especially from adults who are doing something they don't want their kids to do. That's all fine and dandy, but does it really work? I'd have to say **NO,** it doesn't work as well as adults/parents like to think.

A perfect example is babies. From the minute they are born, they are looking and observing. It will be a couple years or so before they can talk, but their sense of observation is strong and keen. Every parent looks on in amazement the first time their child does something they didn't think they knew how to do: turn on a television, open a door, put toys in the toy box, etc.

It's in our nature to observe and do what we see around us, especially those close to us. As the child gets older, he will continue to emulate those closest to him, especially his parents.

We all know that many teenagers often go through a rebellious stage and try to find their own identity, but even then they will still have some of the habits and mannerisms they were taught by their parents. Some good, some bad. This is where Family Fitness is especially important.

It's important to instill a healthy lifestyle BEFORE kids become teenagers. It's vital to get them into healthy habits early so it's ingrained into their psyche. So when they enter those teenage years and start to think they know EVERYTHING and those older than them know NOTHING, their transition to adulthood won't be so turbulent.

On the flipside, if a child wasn't exposed to a healthy upbringing, they may have a tougher road to travel as they get older. According to the Alabama Coalition Against Domestic Violence:

1. Family history of violence, sexual abuse by a female, maternal neglect, and lack of supervision were all associated with a threefold-increased risk that the abused would become an abuser.

2. A child's exposure to the father abusing the mother is the strongest risk fact for transmitting violent behavior from one generation to the next (American Psychological Association, Violence and the Family: Report of the APA Presidential Task Force on Violence and the Family, 1996)

3. According to the Department of Criminal Justice, nationally, 7.3 million children have at least one parent in jail or prison. Sadly, 70% of these kids are doomed to follow in the same footsteps as their parents, becoming imprisoned at some point in their lives. In fact, children of incarcerated parents are five times more likely than their peers to commit crimes. However, these at-risk children are largely ignored before they get into trouble.

There are many, many books and years of research that echo the statistics above. The purpose of this book isn't to go into detail about these situations, but for us all to be aware of how strong an influence parents have on their kids.

Parents hope their kids don't pick up their bad habits, but in countless studies they do.

Also, keep in mind that a parent's negative influence does NOT mean that child will follow in their footsteps. Many children have overcome rough childhoods to become healthy, productive adults. But at the same time, it's up to the parents to give their children a healthy, positive environment to live in.

There are many positive examples of children following in their parent's footsteps.

In the sports world:

Ken Norton Sr.
Professional boxer known for legendary fights against Muhammad Ali

Ken Norton Jr.
Pro football player who won 3 consecutive Super Bowls (92-94)

Rick Barry
Won an NBA championship in 1975 and was named the MVP

Brent Barry
Won the NBA Slam Dunk Competition in 1996 as well as 2 championships in 2005 & 2007

Muhammad Ali
Considered by many to be the greatest boxer in history. He's also an icon who was opposed to the Vietnam War.

Laila Ali
She is the greatest female boxer ever. She holds a record of 24-0 with 21 KO's in her nine-year career.

Dale Earnhardt
He won 76 races and his seven Championships are tied for the most with Richard Petty

Dale Earnhardt Jr
He won 18 races.

Archie Manning
He led the league in passing yards and completions in 1972

Peyton Manning
He was elected to the Pro Bowl eight times, has led the league in touchdowns for three seasons and held the highest passer rating for three straight seasons (2004-2006). He was also the Super Bowl MVP in 2006.

Eli Manning
He's Peyton's younger brother and won 2 Super Bowls with the New York Giants.

This is just a small sample of father-child pro athletes. Others are Yannick Noah and Joaqhim Noah, Tim Hardaway Sr. and Jr., and Richard Petty and Kyle Petty.

Then there are the entertainers:

Actor Tony Curtis and daughter Jamie Lee;

Singer and actor Billy Ray Cyrus and his daughter Miley Cyrus;

Musician Pete Escovedo, an Afro-Latin American musician, father of

Sheila Escovedo, AKA Sheila E, and brother of Coke and Alejandro Escovedo (also musicians);

Filmmaker and TV news producer Sy Kravitz and actress Roxie Roker, who played on "The Jeffersons", were the parents of musician Lenny Kravitz;

Lenny and his former wife Lisa Bonet are the parents of actress Zoe Kravitz;

Musician Bob Marley was the father of musicians Ziggy, Julian, Ky-Mani, Stephen, Damian and Rohan Marley;

This is just a (very) small sample of children who followed in their parents' footsteps.

There are also many instances of children following their parents into other professions such as the military, the family business, medicine, and other professions.

Many of us know someone who followed the same career path as their parent(s). I personally know of a woman who became a doctor like her mother, and a gentleman who became an ordained minister like his father.

Please note: This does NOT mean that kids of pro athletes and other professions are destined to choose the same profession as their parents.

There are many kids who have not followed in their parent's footsteps and choose their own path instead. But at the same time, a parent's influence on their child cannot be denied, and that's the point I'm trying to make.

It's important that we as parents (and others in a role of influence) lead by example and let them see someone being successful first hand, as opposed to hearing about it second hand or reading about it on the Internet.

As far as "success," that is purely subjective. For example, my mother wasn't famous. She never made the news or had anyone ask for her autograph. But to ME, she was a success: she graduated from college. She taught in the Chicago Public School system for over 20 years. She got up every day and went to work. She kept a roof over our head.

I remember seeing her get ready for work, wearing her nice business clothes, carrying her schoolwork in a briefcase.

She raised me by herself on the south side of Chicago and kept me safe and out of trouble. She taught me how to do basic housework (even though I hated it) and how to take care of myself. When I was younger, in my teen and preteen years, I didn't understand what she was doing or why she worked so hard. I didn't understand why she was so tough on me.

But now that I'm older and "get it," I understand now what she was doing, and NOW I can fully appreciate what she did and how great she was. It wasn't about money or fame and prestige. It was just her being her and doing what she had to do for us to survive!

A person can be successful in many different ways and this is just one example that I saw firsthand. The success I'm referring to can't be bought. It must be shown and lived. A big mistake many people make is to tell their kids to live one way, yet they themselves aren't living that way.

Remember: Kids are very visual. They pick things up based on what they see.

Using smoking as an example, according to Medical News Today, 12 year olds whose parents smoked were more than two times as likely to begin smoking cigarettes on a daily basis between the ages of 13 and 21 than were children whose parents didn't use tobacco.

Parents must accept the fact that their kids WILL pick up some of their habits. Some good, some bad. No one knows which habits they'll pick up, but it's inevitable. None of us are perfect. We ALL do things we shouldn't, or have bad habits that we'd like to break or don't want our kids to pick up.

No parent wants their child to pick up their bad habits, so it's important to balance out those bad habits with something good.

Personally, I'm a smart phone addict. I'm almost always using my phone in some capacity. I can't seem to go very long without using my phone! I do the majority of my activities on my phone: pay bills, surf the Internet, research, check email, etc.

I even wrote this entire book on my phone.

I check it while at stop lights, watching TV—any and everywhere! My son sees this and I know he's going to pick up this habit. No matter how much I tell him not to, I know my actions will carry more weight than my words and he'll probably pick up this bad habit.

So, with that said, it's important that I give him some good qualities to emulate as well!

Thanks to the media, kids are constantly bombarded with negative images. Images of violence, sex, lack of morals, etc. are easily accessible to kids of all ages. Unfortunately, parents may not even realize what their kids have been exposed to, so it's even more important that they expose them to something positive on a consistent basis.

Telling your child *"Don't do what I do"* while not giving them a positive alternative to follow may be doing more harm than you realize.

Some of the most powerful, positive influences in a child's life don't require money or a lot of material items.

Ask yourself: What lessons or values would you have liked to have received from your parents when you were a child that money couldn't buy?

And for the parents: What qualities could you teach your child that would last them a lifetime?

There are many things that can be done on a daily basis that cost no money. Things children can experience firsthand:

Hard work
Strong work ethic
Patience
Optimism
Principals
Healthy eating habits
Exercise and fitness
Importance of education (school or trade)
Self-reliance
Self-acceptance
Tolerance of others
These (and many others) are all things that are best shown to a child as opposed to being told about. A child seeing these principals applied on a daily basis will also learn how to not only use them when they are older, but hopefully pass them on to their children.

As said before, children have a mind of their own and may stray away from your teachings, but it's a parent's responsibility to give them the tools to be productive citizens. All we can do is show them the way and hope they follow that path.

WHERE WE STAND

An important part in a child's development is keeping them physically active.

According to the CDC, childhood obesity has more than doubled in children and quadrupled in adolescents in the past 30 years.
The percentage of children aged 6–11 years in the United States who were obese increased from 7% in 1980 to nearly 18% in 2012. Similarly, the percentage of adolescents aged 12–19 years who were obese increased from 5% to nearly 21% over the same period.

In 2012, more than one third of children and adolescents were overweight or obese. Overweight is defined as having excess body weight for a particular height from fat, muscle, bone, water, or a combination of these factors. Obesity is defined as having excess body fat.

Overweight and obesity are the result of "caloric imbalance"—too few calories expended for the amount of calories consumed—and are affected by various genetic, behavioral, and environmental factors.

There are many factors why the obesity rates for our young people are rising, but there's one reason I take as a personal offense: When I was growing up in the '70s and '80s, we played OUTSIDE. Punishment for us was keeping us inside! Many kids nowadays prefer to stay inside to play, but for me and my peers, we were ALWAYS outside.

We rode our bikes; played Hide & Seek; played on the swings, monkey bars etc.; and we walked to the park and played football, baseball, or basketball. I also remember watching the girls jump Double Dutch every day.

Going outside was our JOB. We woke up, ate breakfast, asked if we could go out, and off we went! Home for lunch then back outside. "Quitting time" was when the street lights came on. Then it was time to go home! I can remember very clearly my friends knocking on the door asking if I could go outside and the sheer JOY of putting my shoes on and going out to play!

Kids nowadays don't do that, or not to the extent we did years ago. Many kids PREFER to stay indoors, as that's where all their toys are:

Video games
Flat screen TVs
Cable/satellite TV
Etc.

According to the President's Council on Fitness, Sports, and Nutrition, children now spend more than seven and a half hours a day in front of a screen (e.g., TV, videogames, computer). Punishment for the average kid today is to TAKE AWAY their electronics.

Many would be quick to say that this is why so many of our kids are overweight: the lack of physical activity and too much time playing video games or sitting in front of the TV is the cause. While this may be true, there are other factors that must be taken into account.

The world has changed quite a bit since I was a kid. As I said before, we'd be outside hours at a time, coming home only to eat. For several hours at a time, my mother knew I was outside, but didn't know EXACTLY where I was. She had a general idea, but didn't know my exact location. Today you might be hard pressed to find a parent who will let their kids out of sight (or hearing distance) for a very long time...

Is there a rise in the crime rate? It depends on who you ask. Violence and crime has always been a problem, but we hear more and more stories of kids getting abducted and harassed today than in years past. This might be in part to how fast we can obtain information now thanks to the Internet, but it's enough to scare many parents and prompt them to keep a close eye on their children.

And I don't blame them one bit.

Whatever the reason, kids aren't outside playing like previous generations. Then there's the fact that many schools across the nation are cutting back on gym classes.

According to ABC news, gym classes are being sacrificed across the country to save money and satisfy federal mandates stressing test scores in math and reading. A little more than half of students nationwide are enrolled in a physical education class, and by high school only a third take gym class daily, according to the National Association for Sport and Physical Education.

And it's not like most kids are making up for lost gym classes by working out on their own time. More than 60% of children ages 9 to 13 do not participate in any organized physical activity during their non-school hours, the Centers for Disease Control and Prevention reported in August 2013. And 23% do not engage in any free-time physical activity at all.

Translation: Fewer kids are playing outside.

The statistics are troubling. According to a 2012 report from the American Medical Association, among young people ages 6 to 19:

Obesity Rates of American Children
Ages 6-19

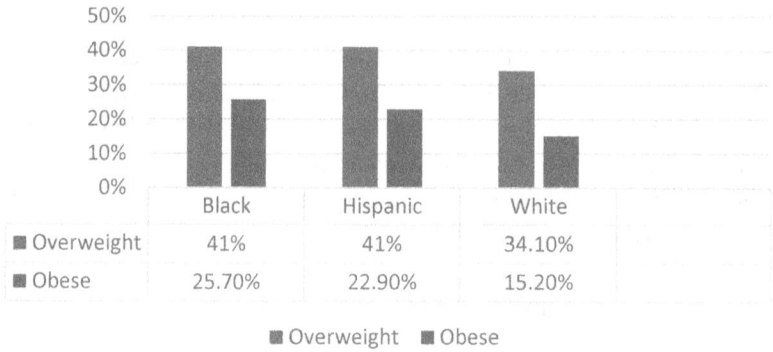

	Black	Hispanic	White
■ Overweight	41%	41%	34.10%
■ Obese	25.70%	22.90%	15.20%

■ Overweight   ■ Obese

- Almost 1 in 3 (33.2%) are considered to be overweight or obese, and 18.2% are considered to be obese.
- More than 2 in 5 black and Hispanic youth (more than 41%) are considered to be overweight or obese.
- About 25.7% of black, 22.9% of Hispanic, and 15.2% of white youth are considered to be obese.

This extra weight can have serious health consequences. Obese children are at risk for a number of conditions, including:

High cholesterol
High blood pressure
Early heart disease
Diabetes
Bone problems
Skin conditions such as heat rash, fungal infections, and acne

I find these statistics quite offensive. Kids aren't going outside to play, gym classes are being cut, and as a result, our kids are at an increased risk for diseases that they shouldn't have to worry about until decades later.

But wait. There's more: We eat too much fast food. According to a policy brief by the UCLA Center for Health Policy Research in 2013, a large percentage of very young children in California, including 70% of Latino children, eat fast food regularly.

The study found that 60% of all children between the ages of 2 and 5 had eaten fast food at least once in the previous week.

The majority of the state's young children also do not eat enough fruits and vegetables, with only 57% of parents reporting that their child ate at least five fruit and vegetable servings the previous day.

These are statics from California, but this is not just a California problem.

These numbers are very troubling. There are many reasons (in my opinion) why we're eating so much fast food, thus getting larger as a society:

More than 23 million Americans, including 6.5 million children, live in "food deserts"—areas that are more than a mile away from a supermarket. Since the 1970s, the number of fast food restaurants has more than doubled.

Not only is it easier to get fast food for some than it is to get healthy foods, it's also CHEAPER to purchase in many cases. A person can purchase a value meal that consists of a burger, fries, and a soda in one convenient stop. They don't even have to get out of their car.

Most grocery stores don't have that type of convenience.

A person can buy a pack of hotdogs, frozen pizza, etc. for literally a couple dollars. When I was struggling and in between jobs, I would go to the store and buy a pack of hot dogs and white bread for $2.00 and change. Why? Because it was so cheap and easy. Did I want to eat hot dogs and white bread? Absolutely not, but when you're barely getting by you may not have a choice.

In my experience, the healthier foods were more expensive. A great example is organic food. Organic food can be very pricey, and a person may want to eat healthier, but simply can't afford it. Many will disagree with that, but my personal experience says otherwise.

Another reason is the simple fact that fast food is just that: FAST. How many people reading this have families? How many people reading this work 8-10 hours a day, and don't have either the time or energy to cook after a hard day's work? For many (especially single parents), their day doesn't end when they leave work; it's just beginning:

Some must rush to pick up their kids from day care, or others are taking them to baseball or karate practice. Eventually, they'll get home to help the kids with homework. Finally, it's time to get them ready for the bed.

This is the life of many parents across the country. Day after day, week after week, month after month.

It seems we are busier and busier, and some don't have the time (or energy) to cook healthy meals on a consistent basis. So seeing how that fast food restaurant is on practically every corner, it's too easy and simple to hit the drive thru and pick something up.

It's not about being right or wrong, it's the reality some people live in this day and age. Unfortunately, this reality is wreaking havoc on our health. Parents are too busy to cook, kids don't understand that the fast food isn't good for them (even though it tastes good), and they are being taught bad eating habits that will follow them into adulthood.

Looking at the statistics above, things aren't getting better, they're getting worse.

So when you tie everything together (lack of exercise, sitting in front of the TV or computer for hours at a time, and eating fast food), our kids health is in serious jeopardy.

They don't know any better, but we adults do. It's up to us to show the next generations how to live a healthy lifestyle. Decades from now, our kids will be the leaders of this country, and also taking care of their parents (us). The worst case scenario is if these trends continue, they will barely be able to take care of THEMSELVES, let alone the COUNTRY, because they'll have the same ILLNESSES as their parents.

This is something that must be addressed but it's not talked about like it should be.

Another aspect that must be addressed is the importance of education and our ability to compete with other nations. As the economy becomes more and more global, it's crucial that our kids have some type of education or skill that will provide them with the ability to take care of their families.

In the '50s and '60s, there were many factory jobs a person could get right out of high school where they made a decent salary and could work there until retirement age. Over the years, many of those jobs relocated overseas for a variety of reasons, but the end result is those jobs are not on US soil.

Using the clothes on your back as an example, where were they made? How about the shoes on your feet? Many of these items used to be made in the US, but they are not anymore.
Instead of working at a factory like their great grandparents, many kids of today (and the future) will be forced to work in fast food or a call center. These jobs pay low wages and make it very difficult to have a decent standard of living.

Education is the key, be it a college degree or a skill that demands a higher salary. The importance of education is becoming more and more important as the years go by, but it seems to be taking a back seat:

In 2013, the US ranks 24th in literacy:

According to the Program for International Student Assessment, the average reading literacy score for 15-year-old American students is 498 (out of 1000 possible points). That is enough to make the United States rank twenty-fourth out of sixty-five educational systems ranked in that category. Shanghai, China, ranked first, with a score of 570.

2013 Global Reading Rankings

570	542	545	536	512	498	483	477	
SHANGHAI-CHINA	SINGAPORE	HONG KONG	KOREA	NEW ZEALAND	UNITED STATES	SWEDEN	GREECE	

■ Mean Score

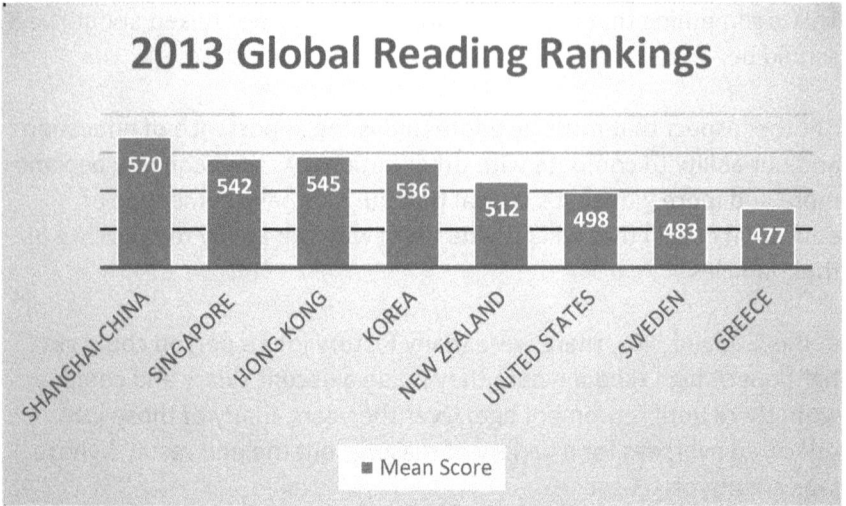

The U.S. ranks 14th in educational performance:
According to the report, The Learning Curve, developed by the
Economist Intelligence Unit, the United States ranks fourteenth out of
forty countries ranked in overall educational performance. South Korea
ranks first. The top ten countries in educational performance are:

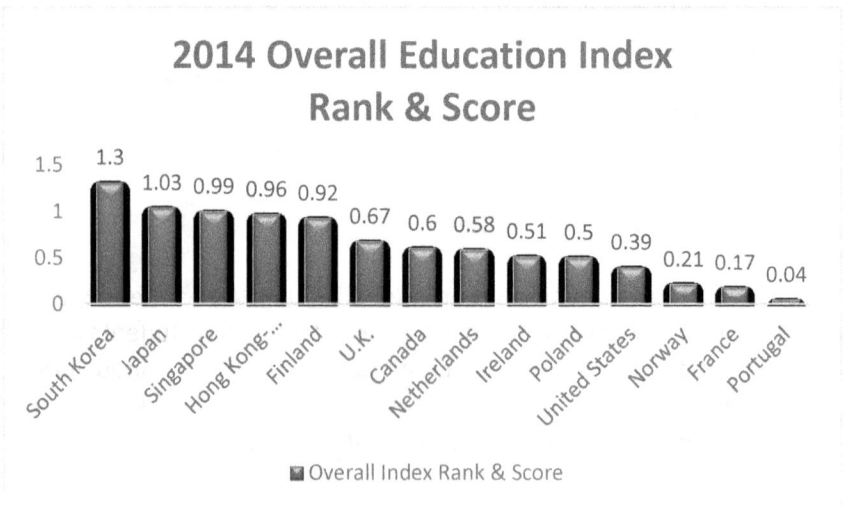

2014 Overall Education Index
Rank & Score

South Korea	Japan	Singapore	Hong Kong...	Finland	U.K.	Canada	Netherlands	Ireland	Poland	United States	Norway	France	Portugal
1.3	1.03	0.99	0.96	0.92	0.67	0.6	0.58	0.51	0.5	0.39	0.21	0.17	0.04

■ Overall Index Rank & Score

In 2001, U.S. students finished 15th in reading, 19th in math and 14th in
science—in a study that only ranked 31 nations.

In 2006, the US ranked 33rd in reading, 27th in math, and 22nd in science.

Many people will question the accuracy of these tests and say the numbers are incorrect. I will leave the exact ranking for others to debate, but what I'm looking at are the trends.

In yet another study, "The Economic Impact of the Achievement Gap in America's Schools," it is noted that in the 1950s and 1960s America led the world in K–12 education just as we led the world with our economy.

No matter what study you look at today, we are NOT #1, and that's what's most important.

"With high levels of youth unemployment, rising inequality and a pressing need to boost growth in many countries, it's more urgent than ever that young people learn the skills they need to succeed," said The Organization for Economic Co-operation and Development (OECD) Secretary-General Angel Gurría. *"In a global economy, competitiveness and future job prospects will depend on what people can do with what they know. Young people are the future, so every country must do everything it can to improve its education system and the prospects of future generations."*

When I worked as a financial advisor, we were taught to pick stocks by looking at trends and forecasts. We didn't choose stocks based on what they were doing in the present, but for what they could possibly do in the future. We couldn't predict the future of course, but we would use various data to find the best investments for our clients. Using that same philosophy, I find these trends very troubling.

Our children (on average) aren't getting enough exercise. They're larger than previous generations, and we are lagging behind other nations in terms of education. Many of our young people are falling victim to illness and diseases that their grandparents might experience.

So, I ask you: How productive will they be if they're suffering from the effects of diabetes, high blood pressure and other illnesses at an early age? In order for our country to remain competitive and a global superpower for decades to come, we need strong, able-bodied, healthy and intelligent young people in control.

The statistics say many of our young people will NOT meet this criteria.

Many will dismiss what I'm saying and that's fine. They will say it's not as bad as things appear and that everything will work out.

That might be true, but the purpose of this section is to get people to talk about the future of our young people and what WE can do to make sure they are equipped to be positive, productive citizens.

Instead of dwelling on the (perceived) problems that I personally think are very real and just complaining, it's crucial that we focus on solutions!

The very first thing we must do is take responsibility for our young people, especially parents. We can't expect or rely on someone else (e.g. the government) to help us. We can't count on programs like after school programs or initiatives to help our kids exercise more or eat better.

As government budgets get tighter and tighter, many programs are cut, and among the first to get cut are programs designed to help children and the poor. Short term, this may save the country money, but long term, it may COST the government money in many ways.

While society may be looking at things from a short term perspective, it's up to US to focus on the long term. Our kids need us to look out for their future. It's time we STOP waiting on someone else to take care of things. We have to do it one day, one child at a time.

EATING AND EXERCISING TOGETHER

In previous segments we illustrated how children often take on their parents' habits, both good and bad.

As parents, we prefer they only take our good habits, but that may not be realistic. One habit that needs special attention is our eating habits. What we eat, we will more than likely feed our kids.

So if our eating habits aren't the best, there's a strong chance theirs won't be either. Obesity could soon be a problem for both parent and child. Children whose parents are overweight or obese are at higher risk for becoming obese themselves, studies have shown. A study in the Journal of Pediatrics, for instance, found five independent risk factors for childhood obesity. The main risk factor was parental weight.

Obesity is a major problem in both adults and children alike, and in order for things to change, people must make a conscious effort to make the changes themselves. In addition to eating healthy meals together, it's also a great idea for parents to exercise with their kids.

When trying to make major lifestyle changes, family can be a great support system. This would be a great opportunity for the family to bond by embarking on this journey together where they may not otherwise.
As discussed in previous sections, changing your diet is essential to being fit. In addition to healthy eating, exercise **must** be included in your new lifestyle.

All this sounds well and good, but we have to be realistic. When it comes to the family exercising together, there are some major pitfalls that must be acknowledged:

Scenario I: Conflicting schedules. Mom works. Dad works. Kids are in school.

In a case like this where everyone can't get together at the same time, there may be days where some family members work out together and they report back to the others who couldn't participate.

A great way to make it challenging is to create teams in the family. (Mother and son, father and daughter, parents vs. kids, etc.) Whichever family members can work out together the most, will be on a team together.

Create a family journal or log. All members of the household can write down what they did for the day or week for the others to see.

Have a contest and whichever team wins, gets a prize: new shirts, treated to a movie, etc.

Make it fun! Exercise doesn't have to be a chore or something to dread. Taking care of yourself is serious business, but you can still make it fun. Sometimes a little friendly competition is good!

Scenario II: Single mother who's too busy and too tired to work out.

I have worked with single mothers and I totally understand how much of a challenge it is to juggle keeping a roof over their heads, working full-time, and raising children.

People will say, "Just work out," but for some it really isn't that easy. They may be too tired to work out. I'd be lying if I said I never missed a workout because I was too tired from chasing my 2-year-old around. Kids change EVERYTHING. So to not acknowledge it being difficult for some single mothers to work out, isn't very realistic.

In this situation, heathy eating is crucial. What you eat is just as important as what you are NOT eating.

For example: If you eat an apple instead of a cupcake that will be less calories and more nutritious for you. You'll never hear someone say they gained 20 pounds eating apples (unless they're covered in caramel)!

If you're not working out, make a conscious effort to watch what you eat even more, as the empty calories will add on the pounds.

With that said, there are still ways a single mother can get exercise:

Do you take your son to baseball practice? Daughter to gymnastics? What do you do while you're there? Grab some headphones and walk for 30 minutes. It'll help you clear your mind AND give you a little "me time." Many may not consider walking an exercise, but it's one of the best things a person can do, especially if you're tired or pressed for time.

Can't afford to put them in classes? Grab a Frisbee. Play catch. Play a fun game of "It." Your child will love it and so will you!

Scenario III: Younger kids.

If your kids are preschool aged or younger, they probably have a lot of energy. Take them outside and let them run around as you follow behind them.

If you can take them to a park, great, if not, the neighborhood will do. Most kids are just happy to be able to run out in the open.

After 20-30 minutes you will see that you got a nice workout!

Getting the kids out for 30 minutes or so is great for both of you. It helps them burn some energy (and calories) and you get some exercise in an unorthodox way.

Jogging Stroller and bikes: These are great ways to get exercise and fresh air. Thirty minutes, 3 times a week is a great start on your fitness journey.

Remember: This is a lifestyle. If your kids see you working hard AND exercising, it will rub off on them too.

Scenario IV: Lack of interest: You want to work out, but your daughter doesn't like to.

When dealing with people who don't like to work out, you almost have to trick them into exercising. The key is to find things that are fun that don't seem like exercise:

Walking on a scenic route and just talking. Beach? Nice walking trail? Take lunch and make it really laid back and relaxing.

Riding a bike. Not everyone likes to ride a bike for four hours like I do, but people can ride a cruiser or mountain bike for 30-60 minutes. Find a nice bike trail and get some fresh air.

The plan is to get them to enjoy the other aspects of the activity to the point they'll want to do it again. The plan is they'll associate good feelings with the activity and want to do it more and more. Please note: It might take time, so be patient and be creative with the activities!

Scenario V: Can't afford a gym membership?

The only time I exercise at the gym now is when I go swimming. Other than that, I'm either at home or outdoors. Getting in shape can be as cheap as you want (like buying a $10.00 jump rope) or as expensive as you want (like buying a $2,000.00 bicycle). The choice is yours.

Jogging, walking, and riding a bike purchased from the pawn shop for less than $100.00 can all be done outdoors.
Pushups, sit-ups, and other forms of calisthenics can be done anywhere. When I travel out of town, the only equipment I take are my jump rope and a pair of running shoes. I'll jump for 30-45 minutes and do some core exercises like planks and get a GREAT workout in my hotel room.

Scenario VI: Health issues. Dad can't over-exert himself because of an existing medical condition.

This is a tricky one. If a family member has a medical condition, talk to their physician and find out what they can and can't do. Once the limitations are determined, support that family member by joining them in their exercise program. Let them know they are not alone, and that you all will help them get well by team effort!

It could take months or even years before everyone is on board. However long it takes, don't give up trying to share a healthy lifestyle with your family. These suggestions will only help them, not hurt them.

And remember: Just because they aren't interested right now doesn't mean they won't be later. Be sure to invite them to join in at every opportunity, but if they refuse, don't let that stop YOU from taking care of yourself and having fun in the process. Continue to plant those seeds because eventually they will harvest!

You never know: It's very possible they will see the results you're getting and finally decide to join in.

We all have a responsibility to take care of our families. Don't wait on your husband, wife, mom, or brother to get the ball rolling. Let everyone know how you feel and that it's time to make some changes!

CHAPTER 13: THE BLUEPRINT: SAVING OUR FUTURE

Looking at the statistics I posted, we have no choice but to be more active in our young people's lives. They don't know what they don't know, and that lack of information could hurt them for years to come. They THINK they have all the answers, but most of life's answers are answered by experience. We have the experience and it's up to us to show them the way.

Now I say "show" them because telling people something without the action to back it up is a waste of breath. Telling someone not to smoke while you go through a pack a day is contradictory and people pick up on the hypocrisy. If you say something, back it up with action that they can SEE and EMULATE.

Show them HOW to do what you tell them to do.

Diet and exercise:

It's important to instill healthy habits when children are young. The younger they are when introduced to a new habit, the easier it will be for that child to accept and incorporate it. They won't know any better.

On the flip side, the longer you wait to introduce healthy habits, the harder it'll be as they might be resistant to those changes.

If there is resistance, it's important for parents to remember WHY they are introducing these habits.

1. No junk food in the house.

One of the easiest things to do is not have any junk food (candy, chips, sodas, etc.) in the house. If your children are young, they have to eat what you buy them. If you don't buy cookies, they can't eat cookies. But if you buy apples, that's what they'll eat.

Some great substitutes for candy and other junk foods are:

Yogurt
Dark chocolate
Raisins
Apple sauce
Fruit
Homemade pie made with natural ingredients

2. Show them how it's done.

Kids are very observant. Many will do whatever they see their parents doing, and that includes their eating habits. If you want your kids to eat healthy, it's crucial that you do the same. Leading by example is the key. Let them see you snacking on fruit daily. Offer them a piece of your apple or orange so they can see if they like it or not. Let them see you eating vegetables with your dinner every night.

Also, buy a variety for them to sample as they may like some fruits you don't. I discovered my son likes grapes and apples like me, but unlike me, he likes bananas and watermelon. I like blueberries and strawberries, but he prefers mangoes and cantaloupe. Our fridge is full of various fruits and it all gets eaten.

Let sweets and fast food be a treat, not an everyday part of your diet. When I was younger, my mother wouldn't let me drink soda. It was a treat that I could have maybe once a week. Same with fast food. I didn't like that, because I wanted to eat a burger and fries every day! I used to get jealous of my friends who would eat pizza and other fast food for dinner. It looked so good and they were so happy!

But she wasn't having that, nor did she care about how much I protested. Looking back on it, she instilled healthy eating habits in me because, even though I still like fast food, I can't eat it every day. Too much of it makes me feel sluggish and it upsets my stomach.

Another thing to keep in mind is kids are still growing and developing. Their bodies need heathy foods to grow big and strong. The foods they eat while they're young will either help them or hurt them years later.

3. Tell them how these foods benefit them, and how some other foods hurt them.

Let your kids know what these foods are doing for them. They may not fully understand, but the seed will be planted for healthy eating habits for when they get older.

Many people don't know the nutritional benefits of some of the foods we eat. For example, we've all heard the phrase "an apple a day keeps the doctor away," but do you know why?

Apples improve brain health and diminish the risk of Alzheimer's, lower the risk of respiratory disease, and decrease the risk of colon and prostate cancer. They also have 4 grams of soluble fiber, can lower cholesterol and even clean your teeth.

Not many people know these things, but if you tell a child how good these foods are for them, they might be inclined to eat more of it, ESPECIALLY if they like it!

In order for this to work, it's important that the parents be 100% committed to making it work. That means the parents must eat healthy foods too! As a nation, we are getting larger and larger, so it's not just the kids who will benefit.

4. Tell them WHY they're eating healthy.

They say the only honest people in the world are small children and drunk people.

Kids can be brutally honest. They say what's in their mind whenever and wherever. They ask an honest question and expect an honest answer.

So if your child asks why they have to eat broccoli, tell them the truth. Tell them you're eating it because it's good for you. Tell them the junk food out there isn't going to make them big and strong, but foods like broccoli will. Tell them that it's important to start eating healthy foods now so they will know how to make healthy choices later.

Let them know it's okay to eat that piece of cake, but you have to eat the healthy stuff first!

The earlier in age a person starts eating healthy, the easier it will be for them to make the adjustment. The older that child is, the more difficult it will become. Teenagers can be extremely unpredictable. They may be typical teenagers and give you resistance, but that's what teenagers do! They like to do their own thing!

But how many of us can remember our rebellious years where we didn't want to heed our parents' advice, only to realize years later they were right all along? It's the same in this case. As they get older, they will look back and realize you were laying the foundation for a healthy life. They may even thank you!

Let's just hope they get on board sooner than later!

Also, just because YOU want to make the changes, doesn't mean your children will also. They may be perfectly content eating donuts for breakfast, if they eat breakfast at all. They may even rebel just because they don't want to do what you do, but this is where patience is needed. And when they protest, keep reminding yourself WHY you're doing this. Remind yourself that one day your kids will have to fend for themselves and you won't be there to help them. It's important they learn these lessons now while living in your home, because once they leave, it'll be difficult to monitor their eating habits.

As I said before, it may be difficult, but "difficult" and "impossible" are two different things! It CAN be done, but the key is to be patient. The bad habits didn't start overnight, so don't expect the change overnight. Tell yourself, *It's not "if;" it's "when"!*

Jeffrey White

PILLAR II

MENTAL FITNESS

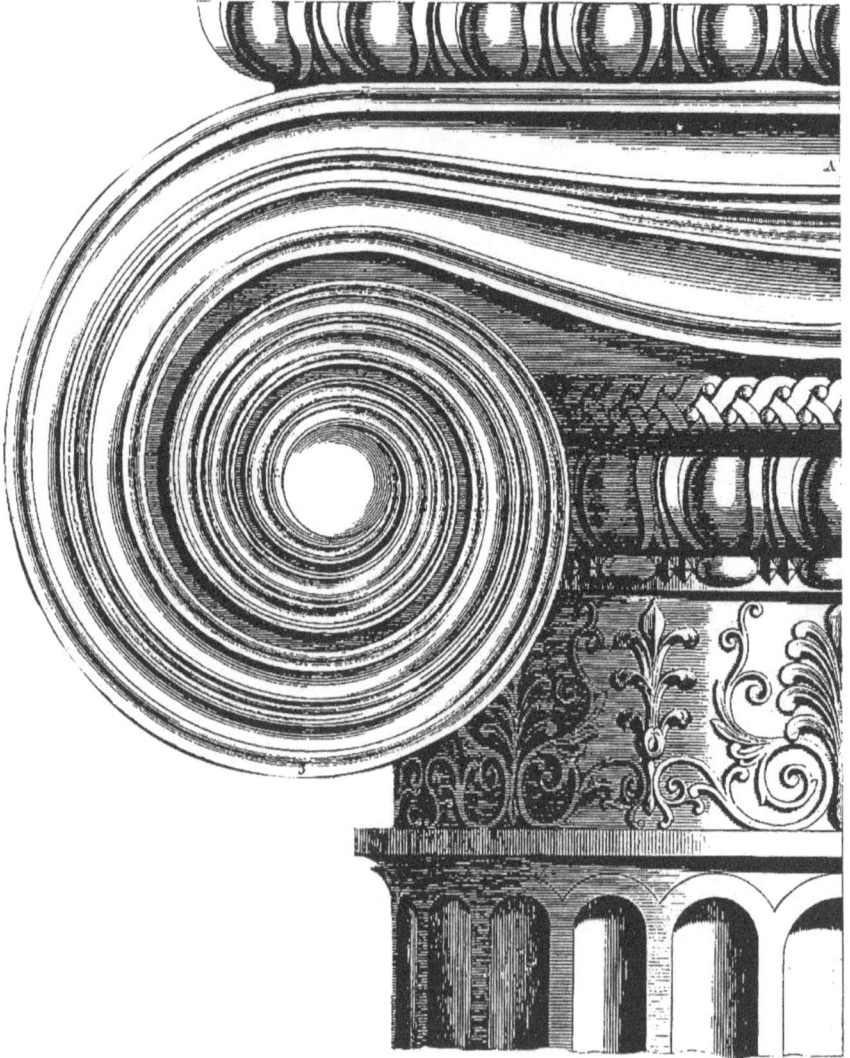

In this section, we will discover ways to deal with life's trials and tribulations and how to overcome them. We'll also give tips on dealing with stress and negativity in a positive way. We will also look at the various ways our bodies react to mentally challenging situations and how our mental and physical fitness can be compromised. Many will debate on which of the 3 Pillars of Fitness are most important, but a person can only go where their mind will take them.

It's time to reach new heights, and being mentally fit is the way to go!

CHAPTER 14: REINVENTING YOURSELF

Life has many twists and turns with many of them hitting you when you least expect it, at the worst possible time. Sometimes there's no rhyme or reason for what happens, and trying to analyze WHY it happened is a waste of time and energy. Instead of dwelling on what happened and why it happened, you just have to adjust and move on.

Here's the scenario:

At age 5, little Johnny had a gift. He was quite athletic and seemed years ahead of kids his age. He was faster than them all!

Five years later, it's obvious that he has a special talent. He can dribble a basketball very well and plays with kids 5 years older than him.

During his freshmen year in high school, he plays on the varsity squad and also plays football and runs track. By his junior year, he's getting national attention. He's heavily recruited by the best colleges to play basketball AND football, but he loves basketball. During his senior year, he commits to the college that won the NCAA championship two years ago to play basketball.

He's a bona fide star his sophomore year in college and decides to leave college and enter the NBA draft.

He's selected #2 in the draft and is now a professional athlete with all the money, fame, and accolades.

Sounds familiar?

Ten years later, our superstar has won two championships and was voted the MVP three times; but, he's lost a step. He's had knee problems and is contemplating retirement. He's not the go-to guy anymore. The new hotshot rookie who grew up idolizing HIM is getting most of the applause, playing time, and product endorsements.

Johnny decides to play a couple more years because the IRS, friends, and excessive spending have wiped out his fortune. He's 31 years old. This is all he knows. He's been playing ball seriously since he was seven.

Two years later, the injuries have caught up with him. He's been cut from the team. He tries out for other teams, but no takers. He's too old and can't play anymore. He's 33 years old and unemployed. Now what?

Sounds familiar?

We all have seen this time and time again. We know this is an aspect of being a pro athlete that can happen at any time. For some, they have a long career, for others, their career is short lived. The NFL is officially called the National Football League, but it's also known as Not For Long.

Either way, we all know it will end at some point for athletes. We just don't know when.

Pro athletes, celebrities, and entertainers can all have similar careers: On top of the world one day, a distant memory the next. A celebrity or athlete can go from *"hero to zero"* in the blink of an eye. It's just the nature of their respective industries.

But is it just their industries?

Scenario #2:

Bob used to watch his father build stuff when he was a kid. Eventually, he started helping his dad build and repair things around the house. He knew early on this is what he wanted to do. While other kids were talking about GOING to college, Bob thought about BUILDING the residence halls they'd be living in.

Twenty years later, Bob is a contractor. Married with three kids, he has his own business and specializes in building new homes. The real estate market is booming. He can't keep up with the demand! He's expanded his business and has a dozen employees. He's making close to $500,000 a year and is living the American Dream.

Suddenly, almost overnight, the real estate market crashes. Home values are plummeting. Many homes are only partially built as homeowners try to back out of their loans. Homes go into default. Bob's revenue drops dramatically. Overnight, he can't afford to pay for his leased equipment. He lays half of his staff off. The kids are oblivious to what's going on, but his wife is worried.

He holds on for another year, but the market is just too bad. The banks seize his trucks and equipment. He's having trouble paying his own mortgage. Angry, frustrated and afraid, Bob files for bankruptcy. Forecasters predict the housing market to be down for several more years.

What's he to do now? This is all he knows.

Sounds familiar?

This is not too much different from the first scenario. In the simplest of terms, they found their gifts at a young age and those gifts turned into a profitable business venture.

In this case, Bob was the owner, player, and coach of the team because he owned the business, hired employees, and told them what to do.

Unlike our pro athlete friend Johnny, Bob could probably start another team when the "fans" want him to "play" again, but it could be years before he gets back on track. In the meantime, he's still in a similar situation as the pro athlete.

Scenario #3:

Kim didn't go to college, but she got a part-time job at the post office in the mail room during her senior year high school. She loved her job and really wanted to excel. Her supervisors noticed and she was promoted to full-time within a year of graduating.

Two years later, she's still doing well. She's been Employee of the Month many times, and was even promoted to supervisor after her boss retired. While her old classmates are either in college or still trying to find their way, Kim has found her niche and is happy. She LOVES her job!

Sounds familiar?

Twenty years later, she's still going strong. She considers herself a "lifer," and is looking forward to retiring from the post office and getting a nice pension one day. Unbeknownst to her, business has been suffering more than she knew. Thanks to the Internet, fax machines and other competitors, profits have been steadily decreasing over the years.

People just aren't sending letters and packages like they used to. Fuel prices are eating away at profits like termites on wood. She saw volume decrease, and heard rumors of layoffs but thought she'd be ok because of her tenure. Not to mention, they had never laid people off before. Never!

Besides, it could NEVER happen to her, not with all the dedication she's shown over the years! One day she comes to work and there's a lot of hustle and bustle in the office. People from the corporate offices are there (unannounced), pulling people into an office one by one.

Kim is asked to come in, and close the door behind her. Kim is nervous, because she doesn't know what's going on. Her immediate supervisor of 5 years is already in the room. He can't look her in the eye. They close the door behind her, thank her for a job well done, but tell her this is her last day. She can get her belongings but must leave the premises shortly thereafter.

Twenty minutes later, Kim is sitting in her car in the parking lot, STUNNED. Twenty-something years of hard work and dedication, GONE. Just like that. This is the only job she knows. No college education, no other experience. Kim feels like she just got slapped in the face.

Sounds familiar?

Like the first two examples, Kim was good at what she did and was getting paid to do it. However, unlike them, she wasn't a star in the beginning. She was a second string role player who came off the bench. But once she was given the chance to "play," she quickly excelled. Unfortunately, the team no longer needed her and she was cut.

Like the others, she now finds herself on the outside looking in, wondering what her next move should be.

Scenario #4:

Kevin was always a smart kid. All his grade school teachers raved about how smart he was. He was teased by his classmates for being a "nerd" or "bookworm," but that didn't stop him from getting straight A's.

It hurt that they teased him, but his mother kept pushing him to get good grades so he could get a scholarship and go to college.

She wanted Kevin and his sister Nicole to go to college, get good jobs, and have a better life than she ever had. As a single mom, Kevin's mom worked two jobs to keep a roof over their heads and to make sure they had birthday and Christmas gifts.

Kevin is on a mission. He sees how his mom struggles and wants to help her out as soon as he can. He's convinced that a college degree will get him that dream job and they all can live well!

Kevin is ranked #3 in his high school class. He gets partial scholarship offers and decides to go to a prestigious, yet expensive Ivy League school. He has to get student loans and a part-time job to cover the balance of the tuition as his mom can't afford to help.

Kevin excels in school. He's going for his finance degree. He decides he wants to work in the business world. Four years later, Kevin graduates with a 3.5 GPA. He has his bachelor's degree and is ready to take over the world! Meanwhile, the country is in an economic slump. Jobs are hard to come by. People are getting laid off and unemployment rates are the highest they've been in 25 years.

Kevin is really confused as he is still looking for a job 5 months after he graduated. It's not supposed to be like this! Three months later, Kevin finally gets a job! He's now a manager trainee at a prestigious bank. Kevin can now use his finance degree. His mom and sister are ecstatic and they all celebrate.

Eighteen months later, Kevin is still working hard. He's putting in 50-60 hours a week working on various projects and visiting different branches to attend meetings and lend a hand. He wears expensive suits and leases a fancy luxury car. He's really enjoying his professional, white-collar life.

Meanwhile, the economy is still shaky. It is announced that his bank has been bought out by a larger bank. The corporate officers of the new bank hold a meeting and assure everyone that business will continue as before and that the bank will be bigger and stronger than ever!

Work continues as usual. The bank name changes, but other than that, everything appears to be the same. Kevin now has aspirations to impress these new bosses and move up as high as he can. Two months later, there's another meeting: branches will be closing and people will be getting laid off.

Kevin receives bad news: His branch is closing and he will be getting laid off. There are no other locations he can transfer to. His career at the bank is officially over. Kevin has a car he's leasing and student loans to pay back.

The banking industry is going through a major overhaul, and Kevin doesn't see a new job on the horizon. What does he do now? This wasn't talked about in business class.

Sounds familiar?

In this case, Kevin trained hard (school) to master his craft (finance). He turned professional several months after graduating college and was starting to hit his stride as he was "cut" from the team.

He's looking for another team to "play" for, but their "rosters" are full. He's stuck.

Each of these examples are all different, yet the same.

Many people look at the pro athlete example and know that happens. At some point, every athlete will have to hang up their cleats. They have to retire and move on.

But the other examples are harder for people to accept.

This happens every day around the WORLD. People get laid off, people get fired, people quit.

The difference is most pro athletes move on. They have no choice. They know the end will come someday. They know they won't be 50 years old catching passes or stealing home plate.

They have no choice but to reinvent themselves. They love their sport, but can't do it anymore. They MUST find a new profession. They may not know when the end will come, but they know that day WILL come.

Now of course there are some who find it hard to move on and that's unfortunate, because they can't relive those days. They're over, never to return. But this same rationale can be applied to everyone else. If you have a job and are getting paid to do it, you are a professional. Whether it's a schoolteacher, janitor, truck driver, or factory worker. You are a paid professional.

Here's where it gets tricky.

As a society, we are told if you go to school and/or work hard, you will become a success. It may take longer than you'd like, but if you keep working hard, the success WILL come. I agree with that logic, but what we're NOT told is how long that success will last in that particular field of choice.

Think about it.

We ASSUME that if we set out to be a banker like Kevin in scenario #2, that our hard work and success means we will have a lifetime of success in that particular field. That's not always the case, ESPECIALLY when you have many external factors that can affect your chosen field.

Many companies are becoming global, and that means the very job you're doing could possibly be done in another location at a much cheaper cost. That other location could be half way around the world.

There's nothing wrong with choosing a career and setting out to be the best and most productive worker you can be, but just like the pro athlete, your career could be OVER much sooner than you anticipate.

This is a reality that many people must face, but may not want to. According to the Bureau of Labor Statistics, individuals from ages 18 to 46 will hold an average of 11.3 jobs. On average, men will hold 11.4 jobs and women 10.7 jobs.

This is NOT what we are told when we are entering the job market. It's the worst kept secret. There was a time when a person could anticipate working at one job for 25-30 years, retire and get a nice pension for the rest of their life.

There was a time when a person could graduate from high school, get a job at the factory in town, and make enough to provide for his family up until they retired. There was a time when a person could graduate from college and be practically guaranteed a nice job upon graduation.

Those days are long gone, and like it or not, the job landscape has changed dramatically. With that said, as the economic market has changed, your mindset must change with it as well.

The statistics don't say under what circumstances a person will have 10 or more jobs, but in this economic climate, it might be safe to assume some of those job changes are NOT voluntary. In other words, you have to be mentally prepared to be looking for a new job at any point in time. You may have a job right now, but no one knows how long you will have that job. Like a pro athlete, your career could be over sooner than later.

 This is where your mental focus and resolve comes into play, because the emotional toll of losing your job and the prospect of starting over can be daunting and intimidating. But this is the world we live in now. You have no choice but to adapt to and be able to change gears at any time.

Some people are able to change and adapt without much strain, while others never seem to recover.

Let's be honest: Losing your job can be devastating, especially if you were a dedicated employee and wanted to stay there. Your whole world can flash in front of your eyes as you find yourself wondering what will happen next, like in the scenarios given above.

Whatever the reason for losing a job, many have a hard time with it because they feel as though they lose a part of themselves, especially if it was a surprise. They lose a large part of their identity. Many people define themselves by the job they have, whether it's the title, the salary, or the perks and prestige that come along with it.

In many cases, this is totally out of your control. It's not your fault your company downsized and your entire department was let go. Many people will become depressed as a big part of their identity is taken from them.

And like some pro athletes, they never get over the fact their career is over, or they're unhappy because they never achieved the level of success they thought they should have. In some cases, they feel their best days are behind them, not realizing that more good days could be ahead if they learn how to reinvent themselves.

In this day and age, we ALL must be prepared for the day to come where we lose our job. Will it come? Not necessarily, but this is a reality that many of us WILL face at some point in our lives.

Very few of us are immune from losing a job. No matter how nice you are, how many hours you've worked overtime, how well you play the game of politics, etc., you can STILL lose your job.

This very scenario has happened to me once and my wife twice. Getting laid off is not fun, especially if you don't see it coming.

Life can be very cruel sometimes. You may ask yourself "why me" or think you have ALL the bad luck, but that's not the case. In January 2013, the U.S. unemployment rate was 7.9%, or 12.3 million people were looking for work.

Once you can accept this bitter fact, you can better prepare for any future changes that might come your way.

The first thing you must remember is you are a PAID PROFESSIONAL, and as paid professional, that means people are willing to pay you to do a particular job. What many of us must understand is the job you're doing right now is NOT the only thing you are capable of doing. Many of us are afraid of change or the unknown, so we prefer to stay in a type of job or industry we already know.

Even if a person isn't happy in that particular field or really wants to do something new, they won't make any changes. We don't want to be taken out of our comfort zone.

Unless they are forced to.

Remember: Just as a pro athlete knows his athletic career will come to an end, your career could very well have the same fate. It's up to you to tap into the skills you have. But how? How do you tap into skills you don't even know you have?

In order to be the best person you can be, you should always make an effort to learn something new.

If your computer had a virus and went to see a computer repair person, and she told you she knew everything there was to know about computers, how comfortable would you be in her abilities if she hadn't picked up a manual since 2003? What if she didn't care to learn?

What if you needed a dentist, and he told you he doesn't need to read any dental books because he learned everything when he graduated dental school in 1981? How comfortable would you be with him as your dentist?

Neither of these individuals would do very well because they are stagnant. Would you feel confident in using them as your computer repair person or dentist? Would you be upset if someone suggested you go see them for help or to get a root canal? Of course you would. You'd think that person was NUTS. They aren't even trying to improve as they think they already know everything. It's just a matter of time before they are out of business.

This same logic applies to YOU. It's CRITICAL that you continuously strive to learn new things. Stay open minded and be receptive to new thoughts and ideas. CHANGE YOUR MINDSET! You are a PAID PROFESSIONAL, and that means you MUST stay abreast of current trends to keep your skills sharp! That does not necessarily mean going to school and getting a four-year degree. There are many ways you can master a new craft.

Years ago I was a financial advisor. Being a stock broker was my passion. I really enjoyed helping people reach their financial goals. I thought I'd do that for the rest of my life, eventually opening my own brokerage firm.

But after the September 11 attacks, my business took a major hit. I was still building my clientele and all of a sudden, people stopped wanting to invest. The markets tumbled and I went several months without a paycheck. I was forced to get a part-time job to get some type of income.

Just like in the wild, it's "survival of the fittest" in the financial industry. I wasn't making the firm any money so I had to go. This was all I wanted to do. I had no desire to do anything BUT to be a financial advisor. Nothing else would do, but I wasn't doing as well as I had planned. To pay my bills, I stayed in the industry several more years, but not as a broker. I worked in the back office, helping other brokers build THEIR business.

I didn't get in the industry to be a back office assistant. I didn't get my licenses to help other advisors build their book of business, but that's exactly what I was doing, and I wasn't happy about it. Not one bit. I had to reinvent myself. I had to come to the realization that my passion was gone, and I wasn't doing what I wanted to do. I gave it my best shot, but it just didn't work out the way I wanted it.

And that's just how life is! Just because YOU want something doesn't mean it's supposed to happen for you, or is the right thing for you. Once I came to that understanding and realization, I was able to move on and be at peace with my short-lived career as a financial advisor.

Am I happy it didn't work out? Absolutely not, but I'm happy that I at least tried and I gave it my best shot! I don't want a life full of *"what if's?"* I don't want to look back on my life and wish I would've tried something, or see a life full of regret. If I had never even tried to be an advisor, I'd always think about it in the back of my mind.

It was an overall good experience, but it was time to put it in my past and move on to the next adventure. But now what? What did I want to do? I was ready to discover my new passion.

Fifteen years ago, if someone would've told me I'd be in the fitness industry and writing a self-help book, I would've told them they were crazy. I was perfectly content and happy being a financial advisor, helping my clients reach their financial goals. I would have quickly dismissed that idea as LUNACY without a second thought.

But little did I know that it would be my new reality, because during that time I had discovered my intense passion for exercise and, specifically, triathlon.

Being a financial advisor is stressful. Very stressful. It's crucial that a person find ways to help relieve that stress so they can not only stay sane, but stay healthy!

There are many ways to relieve stress. Some are good, some are bad. I chose to relieve my stress through exercise. Working out helped me release steam, and I found myself getting in better shape and becoming more and more excited about doing triathlons.

At that time it was a fun hobby, as my true passion was still working as an advisor. It was a way for me to deal with the frustration of cold calling people across the country, asking if they wanted to buy stock from a complete stranger. Running after work was a way to help me forget about the people who said they'd buy stock, only to fake me out at the last minute. While riding my bike and swimming, I was able to clear my mind and think of new ways to meet prospective clients and go over my presentations in my head.

But as time went on, things that were out of my control turned my dream job as a financial advisor into a nightmare. It hadn't occurred to me to try and make fitness into my career. Yet. I was still focused on being an advisor. When times get tough, you don't just quit, you work harder. If people gave up every time things got tough, they'd never accomplish anything. So, I kept fighting. Meanwhile, I was still working out and having fun with it.

It took me getting totally FED UP and at peace with letting go of that financial advisor dream to open my mind up to trying something new. In other words, it took my failure in the financial services industry for me to consider turning my hobby and stress reliever into a new career. I channeled the passion and excitement I had as an advisor into the words you're reading today. It's the same passion, work ethic and desire, just channeled into a new endeavor. We ALL have the ability to change directions. It all comes down to our mental focus and resolve.

What I have learned is life has many twists and turns. Your best laid plans can be blown up into a million pieces, no fault of your own. You can either be angry about it, do nothing but complain and say, "Woe is me," or channel those feelings into something powerful and productive. It can be done. I'm living it now!

So let's look at our previous examples. What could they do now?

Scenario #1:

Johnny is our star professional athlete who is now old, injured, and cut from the team. What could he do now?

Well, Johnny may not be able to play, but he could teach others how to, especially kids. Being a child prodigy himself, he could mentor or train young athletes and prepare them for future professional athletics.

Johnny could coach a team at any level or become an assistant coach. He could start a sports camp for kids. He could become a personal trainer. His name alone could open doors for him and give him new business opportunities. If Johnny changes his focus he will be ok.

Scenario #2:

Bob owned his own business as a contractor, but the housing market took a crash and he's out of business.

What can he do?

Turns out Bob was frugal, and being frugal meant taking care of things around the house and office, which included repairs like plumbing. Bob has decided to change his focus and focus on being a handy man, but on a larger scale. He has solicited hotels, commercial businesses, and private home owners for basic repair needs. No matter the economic climate, if a person's plumbing is bad, they will pay someone to fix it.

Bob has gotten contacts and is slowly rebuilding his business in a new avenue.

Scenario #3:

Kim worked at the post office for years but was laid off.

While working there, she worked in a variety of departments and discovered she likes computers. If there was ever a computer problem, she'd always watch the tech guys come and fix the problem. She would

even work on her computer at home and help repair her family &
friends' computers if they had a virus or spyware.

She has decided to pursue a new career in computer technology and
has looked into taking certification courses, with plans to work in an IT
department. Kim feels comfortable working with computers and is
excited about this new opportunity. She's also considering starting a
computer repair business.

Scenario #4:

Kevin was the up-and-coming recent college grad turned banker. His
bank was bought by another bank and he was eventually laid off.

What could he do now?

Kevin is still relatively young, so he'd be a great mentor to high school
and college students looking to get into the corporate world. Teenagers
prefer people they can relate to, and Kevin would be ideal as he's still
close to their age.

As a banker, Kevin wore nice clothes and understood hard work. He
knew what he had to do to become a success, but circumstances out of
his control derailed his career. With that said, Kevin could teach courses
on how to dress and prepare for interviews. He could teach at a local
college, high school or youth center, explaining what it is like working in
a corporate environment, or maybe become an assistant professor.

Each of these examples are quite doable, but they each have to be open
minded and ready to try something new. You might be happy in your
current job or career, but that may not always be the case. Or you could
lose your job and not be able to find another job in your industry. Then
what?

Whatever your situation, ask yourself: What do you like to do outside of
work? What is your passion? What are your hobbies? What do you like

to do to relieve stress?

If you don't have a hobby or passion, or can't think of anything, start thinking long and hard about it. Life is too short and too valuable to just "get another job" or simply go through the motions. Why not try and do something you enjoy?

In my case, the seed to become a personal trainer and write this book was planted years ago. I didn't know my job at the time was preparing me for what I'm doing now. It's the same with you. You may have no intention of doing anything different, but life has a way of pointing you in a direction you didn't know existed.

Be aware of this possibility and me mentally prepared to go where life takes you!

CHAPTER 15: SELF ESTEEM, STEREOTYPES & THE MEDIA

There are many factors that can cause a person to have low self-esteem. Some of it is from subliminal messages that a person sees over the years and they don't even realize it.

Many of us know young kids are particularly frightened by scary and violent images. Simply telling them that those images aren't real won't console them, because they can't yet distinguish between fantasy and reality. Behavioral problems, nightmares, and difficulty sleeping may follow exposure to media violence.

Children are also sensitive to nonviolent images that can be just as damaging.

Researchers from Indiana surveyed 400 boys and girls between the ages of 7 and 12, of whom 59% were black and slightly less than half were white, to see if there was a correlation between time spent in front of the TV and children's self-esteem. They tallied the amount of TV watched and had the participants complete an 11-item questionnaire intended to measure overall feelings of self-worth.

The authors of the study said that while white male TV characters tend to hold positions of power in prestigious occupations, have a lot of education and beautiful wives, the TV roles of both girls and women tend to be less positive and more one-dimensional. Female characters are often sexualized, and success is often measured according to how they look.

Black men and boys are often criminalized on TV, the researchers said, which can affect their feelings of self-worth. According to the study, self-esteem has significant behavioral and emotional ramifications, and it is often correlated with motivation, persistence and academic achievement, particularly among children.

Young girls are especially sensitive to body image.

A recent study by the Dove Self-Esteem Project (DSEP) in the United Kingdom reveals that a whopping 47% of girls between the ages of 11 and 14 refuse to take part in activities that will show off their bodies in any way — like swimming or performing in a school play.

And 23% are too afraid to put their hand up in class.

Is it possible these feelings were never acknowledged as a child, and as a result have caused a person to sabotage their own dreams and self-confidence as an adult? The teen and pre-teen years are a time when many start to become aware of how they look, wanting to be accepted by their peers, and comparing themselves to the celebrities and famous people they look up to.

Many will want to fit in and be accepted, but don't feel worthy if they don't measure up physically:

"I'm too short"
"I'm too tall"
"I'm too fat"
"I'm too skinny"
"I'm ugly"

When a person thinks negative thoughts, their subconscious mind takes it as truth. Just as a young child believes what they see on television is real, your subconscious does the same.

So, if a person constantly puts themselves down, in time they will internalize those thoughts and start to believe it, even if they put on a happy face for others. These negative thoughts can destroy a young person's self-confidence, and if they are being bullied or teased it will only make matters worse.

This type of thinking could be the root cause of several issues, such as depression, stress or eating disorders.

How possible is it that a young person is depressed due to a bad body image, but doesn't realize that's the cause of their depression? Or their eating disorder was caused by a variety of factors, with one of them being bombarded with images of slender models as the standard of beauty?

As a society, it's important to get to the root cause of the problem, instead of just treating the symptoms.

How many young people are on prescribed medications because of undiagnosed body image problems? How many people are getting cosmetic surgery because they aren't comfortable with their appearance?

It would be easy to put the blame entirely on the media, but we as individuals must take some of the blame also. Magazines, newspapers, the Internet, etc. are in the money making business. Their job is to entertain the public AND be profitable doing it.

In other words, while many of us are looking at it from a black, yellow, or brown perspective, we must also look at it from a GREEN perspective. Ideally, all shapes, sizes and colors would be equally represented in print and on television, but we know that's not the case.

One big reason is because certain images make more money than others.

For example, in China, for a day, a weekend, a week, even up to a month or two, Chinese companies are willing to pay high prices for fair-faced foreigners to join them as fake employees or business partners.

Some call it "White Guy Window Dressing." To others, it's known as the "White Guy in a Tie" events, "The Token White Guy Gig," or, simply, a "Face Job."

The fashion industry has long shunned using models of color. This sentiment was echoed by world famous photographer Steven Meisel: "I've asked my advertising clients so many times, *'Can we use a black girl?' They say 'no. Black girls don't sell.'"*

Hollywood is hesitant to produce more African-American films (one reason is their lack of overseas acceptance). According to unnamed sources, Hollywood executives said when the film *Just Wright,* featuring Queen Latifah and Common, didn't meet expectations and only grossed $21.5 million, it was marketed as a black film. The result was a virtual shutdown of all romantic comedies featuring African-Americans.

George Lucas is arguably one of the greatest producers in the history of motion pictures who made billions of dollars from his *Star Wars* and *Indiana Jones* movies. But even with all his clout, he had a very difficult time getting the backing for the movie *Red Tails*—a movie about the Tuskegee Airmen.

When Lucas approached major Hollywood studios about backing *Red Tails*, he was told, "There's no major white roles in it at all...I showed it to all of them and they said, 'No. We don't know how to market a movie like this'," Lucas told Jon Stewart on The Daily Show.

This is why there is such a push for people to go see a movie when it first comes out, and not wait to see it when it goes to cable or Pay-Per-View. Hollywood is looking at the numbers. If that movie doesn't do well, they won't be willing to invest money into similar movies in the future.

Then there's television, and the important factor to consider is advertising.

Advertising revenue provides a significant portion of the funding for most privately owned television networks (ABC, NBC, FOX, etc.). The vast majority of television advertisements today consist of brief advertising spots, ranging in length from a few seconds to several minutes (as well as program-length infomercials).

The viewership of television programming, as measured by companies such as Nielsen Media Research, is often used as a barometer for television advertisement placement, and for the rates charged to advertisers to air within a given network, television program, or time of day.

In other words, the more popular the show, the more networks can charge for commercials, thus the more money they can make. (The same philosophy also holds true for radio commercials.)

According to Nielson, in 2013 advertising agencies spent $75 billion on television, magazine, Internet, and radio ads, but only $2.2 billion was spent towards focusing on black audiences.

Then there's the advertising rate for 30 seconds on various American TV shows in 2013:

2013 Commercial Advertising Rates

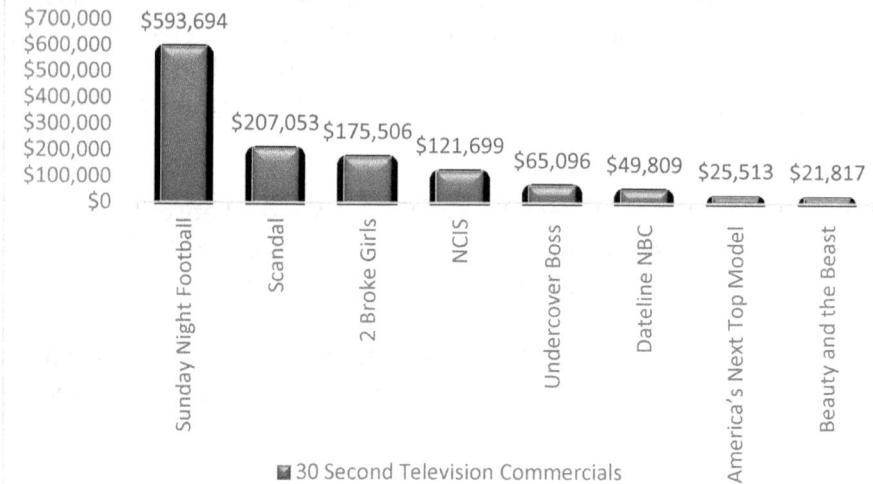

Sunday Night Football $593,694; Scandal $207,053; 2 Broke Girls $175,506; NCIS $121,699; Undercover Boss $65,096; Dateline NBC $49,809; America's Next Top Model $25,513; Beauty and the Beast $21,817

■ 30 Second Television Commercials

Out of the top 91 shows, none were African American shows. This is a very important aspect that can't be overlooked. If a show can't generate advertisers, there's a very strong possibility that show will not be made.

I give the example using African American shows, but the same logic can be applied to any segment of the population that's not being represented on television as often as it should.

Remember: The name of this game is to make money. We live in a society where profits and large bank accounts are a large part of the American dream for many. And that means producing movies and TV shows that will get the most money from advertisers. Companies like Viacom, Warner Brothers and others trade on the stock market, and people will purchase shares of these companies in hopes of making money.

Shareholders demand these companies make a profit, so they do everything they can to make as much money as possible. One way is to create TV shows that will generate the most advertising revenues. If the top 91 revenue generating shows in 2013 did not feature a majority minority cast, then Hollywood may not see a reason to try and create more of these shows.

Instead, they will make shows like the *Big Bang Theory*, which was ranked #3 and charged $316,912 for a 30 second commercial. The public is looking at it from a moral perspective, while Hollywood is looking at it from a business perspective.

A great example is the music industry. Rap and music that promotes violence and disrespects women is frowned upon by many in society, but the record companies keep releasing this type of music because it is extremely profitable.

So now we've come back full circle: Young people don't see themselves on TV and in print in a positive manner, but can listen to a record or watch a music video and see people who look like them doing things that many would describe as illegal, unethical, or immoral.

We also have to take into account how many of the people who look like them on television are on reality shows, fighting, cursing, and disrespecting each other. Or they are the lead story on the evening news where they committed a crime.

If a young person sees this day after day, month after month, year after year, they might think it's something wrong with THEM or that this is how they are SUPPOSED to act. In light of all this, we have groups that will say this is racism and this is just another way to keep people down, but it's much deeper than that.

Racism may indeed be a factor, but it's not the ONLY factor. It's important to support the movies and TV shows that have the images you want to see so they will stay on the air and similar shows can be created. It's critical that people stop watching shows and listening to music that don't help them grow in a positive manner.

While some will argue it's "just entertainment," that entertainment is hurting people in many ways both directly and indirectly.

When people don't see themselves in a positive manner, others don't see it either. While one person is angry and frustrated they don't see any positive images of themselves in the media, the other side could start to believe that's ALL there is to that particular group of people.

The result now is people being judged and stereotyped on what others believe to be accurate information.

For example:

Women:
Very unrealistic goals for ideal body shape make women believe that they are valued because of their bodies and therefore their self-esteem is also based on how they look. The media shows that it is okay to treat women like objects rather than human beings and sends messages to women that by changing their appearance they can get a better life.

Men:
Men, like women, are also depicted with unrealistic body types. It shows men as aggressive and in control, while including women as if they were objects.

Minorities:
African Americans play sports and run really fast. Latinos join gangs. Native Americans drink a lot. Brown skin people are extremely intelligent but easily fooled.

Muslims are viewed as threats and bad people due to some "claiming" that Muslims caused the destruction of people's lives in the bombing of the World Trade Center in New York. Due to this, many people have now changed their views on Muslim people and perceive ALL of them as terrorists, which is unfair. The actions of a select few should not penalize an entire race of people.

Nearly every day in the media they represent Black people (primarily Black males) as criminals and drug dealers. This causes tensions between racial groups and causes some to stereotype and be prejudiced to other ethnic groups.

Blonde hair:
The blonde stereotype has two aspects. On one hand, blonde hair for

women has been considered attractive and desirable. On the other hand, a blonde woman is often perceived as making little use of intelligence and as a "woman who relied on her looks rather than on intelligence." The latter stereotype of "the dumb blonde" is exploited in jokes against blonde-haired women.

Tattoos:
Usually if you see a male who is heavily tattooed, the perception is that they are of a lower class background or lifestyle, that they have probably made poor life choices in the past, and that they are somewhat of a rebel or thug.

This is just a small sample of the stereotypes of various groups that are perpetuated by the media.

The problem is many people tend to believe these stereotypes and treat people accordingly, or those who fit the stereotype suffer from the reactions they receive from others. In both cases, this is detrimental to a person's mental fitness. Relying on the media for your information is a mistake because, as you can see, the media has its own agenda. It is NOT going to show everyone in a positive light or balance out the good and bad.

People say they want more positive images and music, but the numbers say otherwise. Millions of dollars are spent every year on violent movies, video games, music, and sexist lyrics. As long as the demand for these products is high, they will still be produced.

Truth be told, there are good people in all races, ethnic groups and social classes, but you can't rely on the media to give you this information, nor should you expect them to. It is up to YOU to learn the truth. It is your responsibility to not judge a book by its cover, or allow someone to judge you.

It is your responsibility to explain to your kids that they are much more than what the media portrays them to be. It is your responsibility to let your kids know that not all overweight people are lazy and don't exercise, all African Americans are not thugs, and that women are not sexual objects.

Being mentally fit means not letting stereotypes or not seeing yourself in a positive image stop you from reaching your goals. Being mentally fit means that you do NOT stereotype everyone you meet by what you see on television.

Being mentally fit means being proud of who you are regardless of what those around you say, think, or do. You will STILL hold your head high. Being mentally fit is understanding that even though the deck may be stacked against you, it doesn't matter, because you will still succeed in spite of those determined to keep you down!

It's important for a person to get to the root cause of their negative feelings. It's very possible these feelings are the result of some of the examples listed above. If they are, you can start to deal with the issue head on and begin the healing process.

Whatever the cause of these ill feelings, not dealing with them in a positive manner could be detrimental to your health in the form of stress-related illness and the formation of bad habits. It's time to talk about stress.

CHAPTER 16: LET'S TALK ABOUT STRESS

Stress (or the inability to deal with stressful situations) can cause severe damage to a person physically, mentally and spiritually. Being mentally fit doesn't mean you don't encounter stressful situations, it means you know how to effectively handle them.

When was the last time you were in a stressful situation? Last month? Last week? Today? Many of us have experienced some level of stress in the not too distant past, and will probably experience more in the near future.

But what exactly is stress? How can we deal with it?

In its simplest terms, stress is something that causes mental tension. Stress is considered a bad word by some, but not all stress is bad. Some is good, like the butterflies you might feel when you're about to play in a big game, or when you prepare for that big interview. That short-term stress can be good for you. It gets your blood flowing. The stress we need to be concerned with is the bad stress.

Ask yourself: What upsets me? What makes me angry? What's keeping me up at night worrying? This is the type of bad stress we need to be concerned with.

For some, it's dealing with obnoxious drivers or sitting in rush-hour traffic every day. For others, it's a demanding boss, pressuring you to meet an important deadline. Others can't sleep because they're thinking about their bills. Unruly kids, marital issues or other challenges can quickly make a pleasant day extremely stressful and put you in a situation that must be quickly dealt with.

Whatever the cause of your stress, it can be detrimental to your health in many ways.

Long-Term Stress

Here are some of the issues associated with long-term stress, according to health experts:

- Heart problems

- Cardiovascular disease

- High blood pressure (increasing the risk of stroke, heart failure, kidney failure, and heart attack)

- Susceptibility to infections (allergies and autoimmune diseases, arthritis and multiple sclerosis)

- Skin problems (acne, skin rashes, eczema)

- Diabetes (some doctors believe stress causes the immune system to destroy insulin-producing cells)

- Infertility (people who are trying for a baby are more likely to conceive when they're on a vacation or when facing little stress, and fertility treatment is more successful at these times)

These are serious issues and show the importance of keeping stress in check.

Coping with Stress

How do you cope with stress? There are many ways to deal with stress — some good, some bad. Exercise is a positive way to deal with stress, as well as having a hobby like playing an instrument or reading books. Again, not all stress is bad, but negative stress must be acknowledged and addressed properly, in a healthy manner. Unfortunately, many of us are doing just the opposite and are making things worse by eating comfort food to feel better.

Here's a list of some of the most popular comfort foods:
Fried chicken
Cake
Pizza
Hot dogs
Chocolate cake
Chocolate chip cookies
Apple pie
Ice cream

If stress is known to raise your blood pressure, how wise is it eat foods high in sodium such as hot dogs and fried chicken? If stress affects insulin and could increase your risk of getting diabetes, is it possible that cake, cookies and chocolate may do more harm than good?

Understanding Stress

Stress also affects the body in other serious ways. Prolonged stress increases the metabolic needs of the body because stress hormones tend to accelerate heart rate, increase muscle tension, elevate blood pressure, cholesterol and triglyceride levels, and can cause a cascade of other metabolic changes.

These changes increase metabolism and accelerate your body's use of carbohydrates, fats and protein. As that usage changes, there can be a resulting increase in blood sugar and free fatty acids, and protein loss (negative nitrogen balance), respectively.

The increased metabolism can also cause an increase in the use and loss of many nutrients such as vitamins A, C, D, E, K, and B complex, and minerals such as magnesium, calcium, phosphorus, and chromium.

In other words, **negative stress can throw your body out of whack.**

Think of your body as a high-octane sports car, jet engine or space shuttle. In order to perform at its peak level, it needs optimum fuel, and that means eating foods that are rich in vitamins and nutrients on a daily basis. When we are stressed, the body uses even more fuel. As a result, we need to eat even more healthy foods to replenish the nutrients lost during those stressful times.

Stress affects people in different ways, and what one person finds stressful another may not. The key is to know your body, what you consider a stressful situation, and how your body reacts to it. It's important to listen to your body and know when you're feeling the strain of stress so you can protect your body from its harmful effects. This is when your diet becomes a factor.

As described above, stress can dramatically increase the amount of nutrients your body needs, and binging on comfort foods will only make a bad situation worse. Please note: If eaten in moderation, comfort foods are okay; it's when they are the primary source of calories and nutrients that the problem arises.

When it comes to diet and nutrition, we must change our mindset. The foods we eat play a vital role in our health and well-being and. As a result, it's crucial we eat the foods that are designed to help us, not hurt us.

Next time you're stressed, instead of filling up on comfort foods, eat these instead:

Blueberries: Contain large amounts of vitamin C, which, along with other beneficial antioxidants, helps to combat the stress hormone called cortisol.

Low-fat milk: Helps your nerves stay healthy. It can also stabilize your blood sugar, stopping you from feeling those extreme highs and lows when you eat sugar.

Oranges: Excellent source of vitamin C, which helps your immune system function under stress more efficiently.

Brown rice: A whole grain that can help reduce stress. Unlike white rice, brown rice doesn't increase blood sugar and cause fluctuations that can contribute to higher stress levels.

Green veggies: Broccoli, spinach, romaine lettuce, etc., have magnesium—a mineral that helps lower your stress level by keeping you in a calm state.

Sweet potatoes: Good source of iron, which is important for red and white blood cell production. Iron is also resistant to stress, assists in proper immune functioning and the metabolizing of protein.

Water: There's a strong possibility you're dehydrated when under stress because your heart rate may increase and you're breathing heavier than normal. As a result, you lose fluid. On the flip side of binge eaters, you have those who don't eat or drink, thus making their dehydration and nutritional needs worse.

Another negative effect of stress is it can keep a person up at night. Lack of sleep can be detrimental to a person's physical and mental health. Next we'll talk about insomnia.

CHAPTER 17: INSOMNIA: THE LATE NIGHT DISEASE

Even though this topic is in the Mental Fitness section, it also applies to the Physical Fitness section as well. Insomnia can affect a person both mentally and physically, but for the sake of this book, it's entered under mental fitness because of how the insomnia medications and the lack of sleep can affect a person's mental state.

An important part of being physically, mentally and spiritually fit is being well-rested. Even if you don't have trouble sleeping, chances are you know someone who does. Share this section with them as it may help them get a good night's rest.

No matter how hard some try, they just can't sleep. They toss and turn all night, only to fall asleep and wake up a few minutes later. Day after day, month after month, and in some cases, year after year.

There's nothing more frustrating than being tired and wanting to get a good night's sleep, but just being unable to sleep.

Here are some interesting facts about insomnia from the Institute of Medicine:

- People today sleep 20% less than they did 100 years ago.
- More than 30% of the population suffers from insomnia
- One in three people suffer from some form of insomnia during their lifetime
- More than half of Americans lose sleep due to stress and/or anxiety
- Between 40% and 60% of people over the age of 60 suffer from insomnia
- Women are up to twice as likely to suffer from insomnia as men
- Approximately 35% of insomniacs have a family history of insomnia
- 90% of people who suffer from depression also experience insomnia
- Approximately 10 million people in the U.S. use prescription sleep aids
- People who suffer from sleep deprivation are 27% more likely to become overweight or obese
- There is also a link between weight gain and sleep apnea

These statistics show just how widespread insomnia is. But why? Why do so many people suffer with this problem while others don't?

There are many reasons people can't sleep:

Medication. Some antidepressants, heart and blood pressure medications, allergy medications, stimulants (such as Ritalin), and corticosteroids can interfere with sleep.

There are some over the counter pain medications, decongestants and weight-loss products that contain caffeine and other stimulants. As a result, these OTC meds could keep you awake.

Erratic sleeping patterns. Not having a set sleeping pattern can disrupt your ability to sleep. An example would be working a night shift and day shift. Another example is a parent who is woken up every night by a crying baby. She finally gets the baby to sleep, but now she's wide awake or it's time to get up.

These changes could affect your circadian rhythms, which act as an internal clock. Your sleep-wake cycle, metabolism and body temperature are all controlled by your circadian rhythms.

Illness. Arthritis, cancer, lung disease, gastroesophageal reflux disease (GERD), overactive thyroid, stroke, Parkinson's disease, and Alzheimer's disease could cause insomnia.

Chronic pain (such as back pain) could also cause insomnia. It's difficult to sleep if you're uncomfortable or in pain.

Stress, anxiety, and depression. If a person has a lot on their mind, it could keep them up all night worrying and thinking about their problems. They are unable to relax, thus preventing themselves from relaxing and going to sleep.

There could be other reasons why a person has insomnia, but these are the most common.

These causes may not be mutually exclusive. For example, a person out on disability because of illness may be losing sleep not because of health issues, but because their disability may be running out and they can't go back to work. Their situation may be stressing them out, which is causing then to lose sleep.

When dealing with any type of illness or ailment, it's important to determine what's causing the issue before trying to treat it. If you have a leaky pipe, you don't keep mopping the floor or put a bucket down to catch the water and hope the problem goes away on its own. You find the source of the leak and fix it. Insomnia is no different. Once you determine WHY you can't sleep, then you can work to correct the problem.

Many people don't do that. Instead, they reach for the nearest sleep aid to help them sleep

As alluded to earlier, approximately 10 million people are using sleep aides. Some are over the counter, some prescribed. Are these products really helping people sleep? Let's dig a little deeper.

Unfortunately, insomnia is nothing new. People have had trouble sleeping since the beginning of time. Herbs like chamomile, valerian root and St. John's Wort are natural remedies that have been used around the world. Opium was also popular. The Greek God of sleep, Hypnos, was holding a poppy flower. Wine has been a popular choice for centuries as well. It wasn't until the mid-1800s that the first drugs to induce sleep were created.

Bromide and Chloral Hydrate were the first chemical sleep aides, created by German professor and chemist Justus von Liebig. When mixed with alcohol it's also known as a "Mickey Finn," or "slipping a Mickey."

In 1857, Sir Charles Locock created bromide, one of the first drugs to promote sleep and restfulness. It was a very popular sedative and was widely prescribed in the 19th and 20th centuries.

Barbiturates were popular sleeping aids in the early 20th century, but were soon discovered to have side effects and to be addictive. Unfortunately, they could be lethal when combined with alcohol, which also included various side effects, including dizziness, poor coordination and difficulty breathing.

In the 1970s, benzodiazepines were developed as a safer alternative to barbiturates because they had fewer side effects. However, as time went on, benzodiazepines had their share of controversy as well.

To this day, experts still disagree about the mental side-effects occurring in dependence and in long-term use of benzodiazepine drugs. Some doctors and scientists still maintain that the only adverse effect of chronic benzodiazepine consumption is dependence and possible withdrawal symptoms when the drugs are discontinued. Others have found a clear correlation between the poor mental health of long-term users and the chronic consumption of sedatives. The adverse effects usually reported in this context are chronic depression, OCD, phobias, and personality changes.

The FDA was aware of the controversy and in the early 1970s, and they initiated a review of over-the-counter sleep aids in order to find a gentler alternative to benzodiazepines. They approved one chemical called doxylamine succinate, which is an antihistamine that is now found in common cold remedies.

Histamine is a chemical that is released by the body as a reaction to an allergic substance. Antihistamines block the effects of this chemical on the respiratory system, helping to prevent or relieve the symptoms of allergies.

When it was discovered that they also caused drowsiness, antihistamines began being marketed for better sleep as well. If an antihistamine is used for sleeping, it should be used short-term, as our bodies can develop a tolerance to it over time. If you develop a tolerance, you'll have to take more and more of it to obtain the same effects.

According to experts, there is a small risk for abuse, but the big concern here is side effects. MayoClinic.com reports that increased appetite and weight gain may occur. The mucus may become thick and the person may experience congestion. Headaches are another side-effect of these medications. There may be changes in vision. Painful urination and pain during menstruation may be experienced. The American Academy of Family Physicians reports that dryness in the mouth, nose or throat is another side effect of these drugs. Fever, increased sensitivity of the skin to the sun, fast heartbeat, and hoarseness are also side-effects that an individual may experience.

Mind you, all the person wants is a good night's sleep, yet these side effects alone could prevent a person from sleeping. It's important a person knows what they are taking and the possible side effects.

What a person does NOT want to do is start taking ADDITIONAL medications to combat side effects from the one medicine they are taking to help them sleep. In many cases, they may not even realize the sleep aide was the cause of their ailment(s).

I will go into this later, but it's important that a person listen to their body and get to the source of their ailment instead of taking medicines haphazardly to combat their various maladies. You don't want to wind up creating more problems in your pursuit to fix one.

This is where listening to your body comes into play. Being mentally, physically and spiritually fit requires you to be in-tune with your body. Know your body. Listen to it carefully because it will tell you when something is wrong. Not all of your problems may require a pill. Sometimes those pills will cause more problems than you bargained for.

So before a person takes pills, they should take a good look at themselves and ask the following:

Why do I have trouble sleeping?

We touched on this previously, but insomnia is such a widespread problem and it's important to know in more detail what some of the causes are. According to the **American Association of Retired Persons (AARP)**, the following medications are known to cause insomnia in some patients:

Corticosteroids - used for treating patients with allergic reactions, gout, Sjögren's syndrome, lupus, rheumatoid arthritis, and inflammation of the muscles and blood vessels. Examples include: prednisone, triamcinolone, methylprednisolone, and cortisone.

Statins - medications used for treating high cholesterol levels. Examples include: simvastatin, rosuvastatin, lovastatin and atorvastatin.

Alpha Blockers - used for treating hypertension (high blood pressure, Raynaud's disease and BPH [benign prostatic hyperplasia]). Examples include: terazosin, silodosin, alfuzosin, prazosin, doxazosin, and tamsulosin.

Beta Blockers - used for treating hypertension and irregular heartbeat (arrhythmias). Examples include: carvedilol, propranolol, atenolol, metoprolol, and sotalol.

SSRI Antidepressants - used for treating depression. Examples include: fluoxetine, citalopram, paroxetine, escitalopram, sertraline, and fluvoxamine.

ACE Inhibitors - used for the treatment of hypertension, and other heart conditions. Examples include: ramipril, fosinopril, trandolapril, quinapril, benazepril, enalapril, lisinopril, moexipril, perindopril, and captopril.

ARBs (Angiotensin II-receptor blockers) - used when the patient cannot tolerate ACE inhibitors or has type 2 diabetes or kidney disease from diabetes. Examples include: candesartan, valsartan, telmisartan, losartan, and irbesartan.

Cholinesterase Inhibitors - used for treating memory loss and other symptoms for patients with dementia, including Alzheimer's disease. Examples include: rivastigmine, donepezil and galantamine.

2nd Generation (non-sedating) H1 agonists - used for treating allergic reactions. Examples include: loratadine, levocetirizine, fexofenadine, desloratadine, cetirizine, and azelastine.

Glucosamine/ Chondroitin - dietary supplements used for relieving the symptoms of joint pain and to reduce inflammation.

This is very important information. Many medicines have side effects that some of us are unaware of. If you're taking any of these medications, look at your sleeping habits. Are you having trouble sleeping? If so, we may have found the reason why. Taking a sleep aide in addition to the medicines above may be helping you one way and hurting you in another way. It's times like this where it's crucial that you talk to your doctor and let him or her know what you're taking, as mixing medicines can be dangerous.

So if you are taking any of the medications above, ask yourself the following questions:

Are these the best options for me?
Is there something else I can take with less side effects?
Are these to be taken short-term or long-term?

How do these medicines interact with other medications I'm currently taking?

It's important to do your homework. Your doctor can help you, but it's up to you to know what you're taking and how it affects you. Don't rely on someone to have your safety and best interest at heart.

SLEEP & SLEEP AIDES

Before we really get into how sleep aides work, it's important to understand the different levels of sleep and how sleeping (or lack thereof) affects the body.

It seems as though our society has forced many people to squeeze more in a day than in previous generations.

"I'll rest when I'm dead," is a common phrase.

Many don't think about the importance of sleep until they are unable to or don't get enough.

We all know the benefits of exercise and eating healthy, but sleep is just as important to your overall health, and many of our everyday activities can be drastically affected if we don't get enough sleep.

Weight gain: Are you gaining weight and don't know why? Are you exercising and eating a good diet but still putting on the pounds?

Your lack of sleep can be to blame. A lack of sleep can make you feel sluggish and worn down, which in turn can be a sign of a slower metabolism. In other words, your body can't burn calories efficiently when you feel this way.

Stress: Lack of sleep can affect a person's mood and cause irritability. (Do you get cranky when you're sleepy? Sleepy babies are notorious for being cranky.) This crankiness can impair your judgment and in turn add additional stress to an already hectic lifestyle.

Stress itself has many negative effects, but extra sleep may help alleviate some of your stress levels and make you more alert, thus helping you cope with life's issues more efficiently.

Getting sick: Are you prone to catching colds or do they seem to last longer than normal? A lack of sleep might be part of the blame. Sleep deprivation can weaken the immune system, thus making a person more susceptible to colds and the flu.

When we're sick, the body needs extra rest to repair and regenerate itself, and on the flip side, this rest is needed to keep us healthy.

Long-term health issues: According the Harvard Medical School, sleep deprivation over an extended period of time can suppress your immune system and can increase your risk for the following diseases:

Diabetes
High blood pressure
Stroke
Irregular heartbeat
Heart attack
Heart failure
Heart disease

Lack of concentration: It's difficult to focus on an important test, project or meeting if you're sleepy. Adequate rest will help you stay alert and ready for the day's tasks.

As you can see, these are serious issues that could possibly be alleviated by getting proper rest. Getting enough rest is crucial to a person's daily and long-term health.

To elaborate further, there are different stages of sleep:

Stage I: This is when a person is sleeping lightly and can be woken up pretty easily. Eye and body movements tend to slow down considerably. Stage 1 may last for five to ten minutes.

Stage II: In this stage of sleep, eye movements stop and brain waves slow considerably. The heart rate slows and body temperature decreases. Approximately 50% of all sleep time is in Stage II.

Stage III: This Stage is the onset of deep sleep. People are usually very difficult to wake up in this stage, and can feel groggy and disoriented if woken up. Brain waves are a combination of slow and fast waves.

Stage IV: This stage is the continuation of deep sleep. It is very difficult to wake a person up in this stage. (Think of how difficult it is to wake a sleeping baby.) Deep sleep is critical for waking up, feeling refreshed and ready for the day.

Stage V (REM): The Dream Stage. This is the stage of deep sleep where dreaming occurs. Rapid Eye Movements and increased brain activity occurs, as well as occasional twitching in the fingers, face and legs. Interestingly, other parts of the body (voluntary muscle groups) are still.

Personally, I was under the impression that sleep went in one chronological cycle, 1-4, then we start dreaming. In actuality, a normal sleep cycle has this pattern: Stage 1, 2, 3, 4, 3, 2, REM. Usually, REM sleep occurs 90 minutes after sleep onset.

In other words, a person could have 4-5 sleep cycles on a given night. Another point to remember is the type of sleep you get also depends on your age.

The percentage of REM sleep is highest during infancy and early childhood, drops off during adolescence and young adulthood, and decreases further in older age.

Stages 3 and 4 in the first sleep cycle shorten even more dramatically in older people than they do during a typical night for everyone else, so older people get less total deep sleep than younger people do. Also with age comes the lengthening of the first REM stage. Older people commonly enter REM sleep quicker and stay there longer.

Personally, I can survive on 6 hours sleep for a couple days. But if I'm trying to train for a triathlon, I need 1-3 more hours a night. If I can't sleep more, I'm working out less and trying to take a 1-2 hour nap every couple days or so to compensate.

Infants usually require about 16-18 hours of sleep per day, while teenagers need about 9 hours on average. Most adults need about 7-9 hours of sleep per day.

The average person simply needs to get to bed earlier to get more rest. But for some, that may not help them because they simply can't sleep. So they turn to sleep aids.

But before we focus on sleep aids, it's important to understand some important things about sleep. During the deep stages of non-REM sleep, the body repairs and regenerates tissues, builds bone and muscle, and appears to strengthen the immune system. In other words, your body goes through a healing process while sleeping. But don't wait until you're ill to get more rest. Rest is a way to keep yourself healthy and be more productive while awake.

Now let's really look at how sleep aides work and how they affect us.

THE SCIENCE OF SLEEP

Before taking any medications, it's important to know how the body functions, and how that medication will help (or hurt) the body. With that said, it's important to understand not all sleep is the same.

For example, if a person is in a coma or under anesthesia, they are "asleep." But they don't produce the normal brain wave patterns you see in a person who's sleeping normally. Instead, their brain waves are very slow and weak, sometimes all but undetectable.

Sleeping pills are similar, in the fact that they put you to sleep, but the sleep they create is not the same as natural sleep.

It's important to remember that REM sleep is essential to our minds for processing and consolidating emotions, memories and stress. It is also thought to be vital to learning, stimulating the brain regions used in learning and developing new skills. Better REM sleep can also boost our moods during the day.

Human growth hormone is released in pulses during deep sleep, and interruption of this stage abruptly stops its release. (In adults, growth hormone promotes cell repair that is necessary after the stress of weight training.)

Deep sleep is characterized by an increased body temperature, and as perspiration increases, our skin secretes more minerals. Our lungs also breathe out more carbon gas. Our intestines transport more excrements. Our kidneys actively filter the blood. Our organs detoxicate. Our skeleton muscles deacidify. Women menstruate more heavily.

At the same time, over 100,000 billion of cells restore themselves in their 7-year cycle. Growth hormones are released, cells are actively replaced and muscular tissue is built up through protein synthesis. Mineral losses are replenished. Wounds heal. Corticosteroid hormones build up our resistance to infections and tiredness. We become immune again to all kinds of diseases. White corpuscles surround and destroy bacteria. In the lymph glands and the spleen, they remove bacteria from the blood.

Our batteries are recharged again. Released biotin produces the vital hormonal energy that restores our aura. Intervertebral disks regenerate and dorsal vertebrae rearrange.

As you can see, a lot is going on in our bodies as we sleep. This is why we need to sleep. This would explain why some studies show that people who get less sleep have shorter life spans and have other health issues. Their bodies simply don't have time to repair themselves.

The processes that are going on in our bodies can't be rushed. They have to go through their normal cycles. For example, some foods can be cooked in a microwave, but not everything can. Some things must be made in the oven. The same philosophy applies to rest and recovery. A nap is good, but a person must get an adequate amount of sleep to function.

The problem is many people either aren't getting enough, or none at all.

So now, the questions we must ask are these: Are these sleep aids helping us or hurting us? Are sleep aids the answer for a good night's sleep?

Let's take a look.

First and foremost, sleeping pills are to be used for the short-term, meaning no more than several weeks at a time. This is EXTREMELY important. They are only to be used for several weeks at a time, NOT for long-term use!

Here's a disclaimer for a popular sleep aid's website:

"Call your doctor if your insomnia worsens or is not better within 7 to 10 days."

Another says: *"Stop use and ask a doctor if sleeplessness persists continuously for more than 2 weeks. Insomnia may be a symptom of a serious underlying medical illness."*

Another says in the Q&A section of their website:

"Can I take 'xxx' every night?

"'Xxx' is indicated to relieve occasional sleeplessness. Stop use and ask a doctor if your sleeplessness persists continuously for more than two weeks. Insomnia may be a symptom of a serious underlying medical illness."

Most sleep aids seem to have the same or similar disclaimers. One even offered a 60-day free trial, but the underlying theme is the same: Many over-the-counter (OTC) sleep aids are NOT for long-term use!

If a person still has trouble sleeping after 2-3 weeks, it's advised they see their doctor as they may have issues that need medical attention.

For this discussion we will focus on over-the-counter sleep aids.

Unfortunately, quite a few people are NOT going to see their doctor and are taking these OTC medicines long-term. What they don't understand is they may be doing their body more harm than good. It's important to know what medicines you are taking, and how long you can take them.

One potential problem is the longer a person takes sleep aids (as well as other medications) that are designed for short-term use, there's a good chance they will need higher dosages to obtain the same effect.

Alcohol is a good example. The more some people drink alcoholic beverages, the more they'll have to drink to get intoxicated. You obtain a tolerance and your body becomes accustomed to it.

This increased resistance to the sleep aid with a corresponding increase in dosage can be dangerous with sleeping pills, because in time a person may need more and more to get the same effect. In other words, the dosage increases, but the benefit decreases.

When a person becomes used to taking a pill in order to sleep, they will find that they cannot sleep without the pill. What if a person who takes sleeping pills on a regular basis, decides not to take it one night? What if they can't fall asleep? What are the chances they will take it the next night to make sure they sleep?

It's just a matter of time before they are addicted, but they don't know it. They simply want to sleep.

But do they work?

At the time this book was written there were only two studies testing diphenhydramine for insomnia. The first study from the US National Library of Medicine included a comparison of the effects of diphenhydramine (50 milligrams—a typical OTC dose) with those of a placebo in 20 elderly people with insomnia. The participants reported slightly fewer nighttime awakenings with diphenhydramine than with the placebo, but no difference in how long they took to fall asleep, how well they slept, or how long they slept.

The second study, also from the US National Library of Medicine, tested 25-milligram doses of diphenhydramine against a placebo and an herbal preparation of valerian and hops in 184 adults with mild insomnia. Compared to a placebo, diphenhydramine improved sleep efficiency (the percentage of time in bed spent sleeping) based on participants' feedback, but not on automated readings of brain, eye and muscle activity. Neither did it affect sleep onset or total sleep time.

These studies are still ongoing, and it could take years before more conclusive information is available. But one thing that is widely known and accepted are the side effects that some of these sleep aids cause, particularly those with the ingredient diphenhydramine:

Dry mouth
Dizziness
Headaches
Constipation
Urinary retention

Of course not everyone will experience these side effects, but the possibility of one or more of them happening is worth noting.

To make known the risks of these products, the FDA requested in early 2007 that all manufacturers of sedative-hypnotic drug products strengthen their product labeling to include warnings about complex sleep-related behaviors and anaphylaxis and angioedema.

Taking sleeping pills haphazardly has its risks. According to the Substance Abuse and Mental Health Services Administration (SAMHSA), more than 19,000 people ended up in the emergency room in 2010 after taking drugs with the active ingredient zolpidem, a prescription medication used for the treatment of insomnia and some brain disorders. That's about a 200% increase in ER visits since 2005—a dramatic rise that mirrors America's growing reliance on sleeping pills. About three-quarters of the ER patients were 45 or older, and one-third were 65 or older, underscoring the dangers to older patients.

As a result of these concerns, many insomnia sufferers have turned to natural sleep aids like Valerian and Melatonin. Melatonin is a hormone made by the pineal gland, a small gland in the brain. Melatonin helps control your sleep and wake cycles.

Your internal clock controls how much melatonin your body makes. Normally, melatonin levels begin to rise in the mid to late evening, remain high for most of the night, and then drop in the early morning hours.

Melatonin has become quite popular in recent years. It is a hormone that produces a number of health benefits in terms of your immune system. It's a powerful antioxidant and free radical scavenger that helps combat inflammation. In fact, melatonin is so integral to your immune system that a lack of it causes your thymus gland, a key component of your immune system, to atrophy. Melatonin may even have a role in slowing the aging of your brain.

Now because of these amazing benefits people have started taking melatonin supplements in hopes of having the body produce more of the hormone so they can sleep.

Other uses are for Alzheimer's disease, ringing in the ears, depression, chronic fatigue syndrome (CFS), fibromyalgia, migraine and other headaches, irritable bowel syndrome (IBS), bone loss (osteoporosis), a movement disorder called tardive dyskinesia (TD), epilepsy; and as an anti-aging agent, for menopause and birth control.

Other uses include breast cancer, brain cancer, lung cancer, prostate cancer, head cancer, neck cancer, and gastrointestinal cancer. Melatonin is also used for some of the side effects of cancer treatment (chemotherapy) including weight loss, nerve pain, weakness, and a lowered number of clot-forming cells (thrombocytopenia).

How well it works depends on who you ask. Some will swear by it, while others say that it's ineffective and even dangerous. It is noted that some patients experience nightmares, vivid dreams and sleepwalking while taking melatonin supplements.

According to MedlinePlus, melatonin can cause mood changes such as sadness or giddiness, and worsen existing symptoms of depression. These side effects are commonly associated with overdosing on melatonin supplements.

Melatonin supplements may increase cholesterol and decrease blood pressure. Patients with type 1 diabetes have reported elevated blood sugar levels while taking melatonin. Even low doses of melatonin may reduce glucose tolerance and insulin sensitivity. Arrhythmia is often associated with regular use of melatonin supplements.

Studies are ongoing with these remedies and it may be years before we know how accurate they are. In a previous section we talked about trends, and how so many products and exercises have come and gone over the years. Is taking melatonin a trend or something that will be here long-term? Time will tell.

We can't predict the future, but a person should ask themselves if the POTENTIAL for these side effects is worth it?

As a society, we're quick to pop a pill in hopes of it solving all our problems and making everything better. Unfortunately, many of these medicines have side effects that may be even WORSE than what we're taking them for.

Not to mention the potential to becoming addicted to these pills. How mentally fit can a person be if they are addicted to a sleep aid or any other medicine? How physically fit are you if that same medicine has raised your cholesterol level or causes headaches, dizziness or nausea?

The (potentially dangerous) side effects of each medication you take are a real possibility to anyone who wants to take a pill. No one is forcing any of us to take anything. It can be suggested, but no one can force you. It's voluntary in most cases.

But at the same time, there are many who will profit from your desire or need to take medicine. Sleeping pills and other meds are big business:

Worldwide sales of prescription drugs exceed $300 billion yearly with tranquillizers, sleeping pills, anti-depressants and other central nervous system drugs accounting for an estimated $76 billion in sales.

Approximately 10% – 20% of the world population use tranquilizers and sleeping pills with up to 30% of people over the age of 60 years using these drugs (often over many years having been prescribed them at a much earlier age) and who have become "accidental or involuntary addicts."

Now let's look at this from a business perspective.

Many medical companies are for profit, meaning they are in the business to make money. Now the question is, Is that the primary goal? Or is their primary goal to heal people?

The more people who use their product, the more money they make. The less people who use their product, the less money they make. If you owned a business, which would YOU prefer?

Are these medicines really helping you or people getting rich off your dependence on these pills?

People are going to doctors for help and they are being prescribed medicine that is supposed to make them feel better, but that's not always the case. The World Health Organization (WHO) estimates that 33% of diseases today are caused by medical treatment i.e. iatrogenic or doctor induced illness. Doctors are the third leading cause of death in the US after heart disease and cancer, causing an estimated 250,000 deaths each year according to an article published in the Journal of the American Medical Association, July 2000.

These statistics are alarming. They should also make you think.

Before you pop that pill, do your research! Find out what the potential side effects are. Find out if it's addictive and if there's a certain amount of time you should take it before you stop.

And most importantly, look for natural ways to help cure or relieve some of your medical issues. We ALL need to take medications at some point, but the problem arises when we become addicted to those medications. Having an addiction of any kind undermines your ability to become as fit as you can be!

Here are some ways to help a person sleep:

- Take a warm bath before bed to relax.

- A nice massage is a great way to relax and unwind.

- Drink an herbal tea like chamomile, catnip, anise or fennel.

- There is debate on whether this actually works, but give warm milk a try if you're not lactose intolerant.

- Set a sleep schedule. Your body has an internal clock. Once on a schedule, it will adhere to it and get sleep on queue.

- Exercise.

- Meditation. Some people are always "on." They can't stop thinking about what they have to do or worrying about something. Meditation can calm an active mind, thus helping them sleep.

If all else fails, see your doctor.

Insomnia and the inability to sleep will also be talked about in the Spiritual Fitness section as well.

CHAPTER 18: A DAILY DOSE OF MENTAL INSPIRATION

We're supposed to eat a healthy diet every day for our physical health, and that same rationale should be used for our mental health as well. We are bombarded with negative thoughts, images, and people daily. It is imperative that you balance out the negativity with as much positive energy as you can.

When I started working as a stockbroker, they told us to listen to inspirational tapes every morning on the way to work. I was resistant to that idea at first because I preferred to listen to my radio. But as time went on, it began to make sense: If I started the day with positive thoughts, it gave me the motivation to give it that extra "push" and shake off the stress of the job.

The following are 31 (one month's worth) of my favorite inspirational quotes with my additional comments after each. They have kept me inspired and hopefully they have the same effect on you as well.

Choose one and make that your quote for the day!

1. "Becoming the best you possible is the greatest achievement in life." –Unknown
Constantly comparing yourself to others is a sure fire way to feel inadequate or even cause depression and low self-esteem. Your energy should be focused on bettering YOUR life, not worrying about what everyone else is doing!

2. "An entire sea of water can't sink a ship unless it gets inside the ship. Similarly, the negativity of the world can't put you down unless you allow it to get inside you." –Unknown
Work on your mental toughness! Stop LETTING things and people get under your skin. You become upset because you allow yourself to be. But not anymore! Those days are OVER!

3. "No matter how good or bad your life is, wake up each morning and be thankful that you still have one." –Unknown
Today is a new day! Let us rejoice and be glad in it! If you're reading this that means you still have an opportunity to make positive changes in your life. Today is yours for the taking. Claim it as your own!

4. "Ignore those people who're always talking behind your back. That's just where they belong. Behind your back." –Unknown
If a person is smiling in your face and talking about you behind your back, ignore them because they don't have the GUTS to speak to you face-to-face and clear the air! You don't have time to deal with people full of anger, hate, jealousy, or insecurity!

5. "Successful people build each other up. They motivate, inspire, and push each other. Unsuccessful people just hate, blame, and complain." –Unknown
Who do you have in your circle? People who build you up or people who tear you down? More importantly, which person are you? Which person do you want to be?

6. "Be more concerned with your character than your reputation, because your character is what you really are, while your reputation is merely what others think you are." –John Wooden
No matter what you do, someone will have a problem with you. No matter how hard you TRY to mold and create your reputation, all it takes is ONE PERSON to go online and tarnish it, because people will

believe what they want to believe. Don't even worry about all that. Work on being the best person YOU can be, not what people think you SHOULD be!

7. "Even if no one believes in me, supports me or recognizes my efforts, I'll keep going. " –Unknown.
Practically every successful person has been in a situation where the only support they had was the person looking at them in the mirror. The difference between successful and unsuccessful people is the unsuccessful start to listen to the naysayers and believe their efforts are in vain. They think they don't have what it takes. On the other hand, successful people DO NOT CARE what others think! They have faith in their own abilities and KNOW they will succeed, whether others believe in them or not! This is the mindset you MUST have if you're going to succeed. Don't let anyone stop you from striving to reach your goals!

8. "Sometimes I feel like giving up. Then I remember I have a lot of people to prove wrong." –Unknown
This is all too real for me. Not everyone supports my dreams and will tell me in subtle (or not so subtle) ways that it won't work. Why they feel the way they do is not the issue as I couldn't care less about their reasons. Nevertheless, I WILL show them that my dreams WILL come true, and I will THANK THEM for keeping me inspired to keep going when I was ready to quit. When times are the toughest, I will think of all those who doubted me and find that extra strength to keep going! Use those who doubt you as fuel to keep going when times are the toughest!

9. "People were created to be loved. Things were created to be used. The reason why the world is in chaos is because things are being loved and people are being used." –Unknown
Don't let the quest for material items or making a lot of money keep you from valuing and treasuring what's most important!

10. "Those who spend their time looking for faults in others usually make no time to correct their own." –Art Jonak
I'm secure enough to admit I've made MANY mistakes in my past. I can admit I'm FAR from perfect and have a ways to go to become a better person. Am I the only one? Knowing this about myself, how can I judge others for THEIR faults? I'm so busy trying to work on MY issues that I

don't have the TIME to focus on others and their issues. (Nor do I need someone telling me what MY issues are!) We are ALL a work in progress. Stop looking down on others because they have their issues. We ALL have something we can work on. Focus all your energies on improving yourself instead of analyzing the faults of others!

11. "Love yourself for who you are deep in your heart and not for what others expect you to be." –Unknown
You can't please everyone. No matter what you say, think, or do, someone will have a problem with it! Trying to please others will leave you little time to please the most important person in your life: Yourself. Stop trying to be what others want you to be and focus on who YOU are meant to be!

12. "Never get so busy making a living that you forget to make a life." –Dr. Wayne Scott Anderson
It's so easy to get caught up in the rat race when you have bills and family responsibilities. If you're not careful, you'll spend most of your waking hours living to work and just trying to survive. This is NOT the way to live! Don't spend so much of your time working that you don't have any time to enjoy yourself. Don't look back on your life and wish you would've spent more time having fun and doing some of the things you REALLY like to do!

13. "Surround yourself with people on the same mission as you." –Unknown
If you're on a basketball team, you want other basketball players with you, not race car drivers. If you're a surgeon about to perform an operation, you want fellow surgeons in the room with you, not circus clowns and mimes! It's the same with you and your goals. If you're trying to do something positive with your life, you do NOT want to associate with people who have no goals, morals, or ambitions! If the people close to you aren't on the same page as you, it's time to find new friends!

14. "A lion never loses sleep over the opinions of sheep." –Unknown
Lions don't care if the sheep are in the break room talking trash. Lions don't listen to sheep when they tell them they can't do something. Lions go after what they want. Sheep sit and wait for a handout.
When lions **ROAR,** EVERYONE stops in their tracks. Sheep get ignored.

When ONE lion enters the room, ALL the sheep take notice. Lions don't care if the sheep are jealous of their success. If you're reading this, then YOU are a LION. Don't let the sheep stop you from reaching your goals!

15. "Sometimes, you just have to bow your head, say a prayer, and weather the storm." –Unknown

One of my favorite movies is *Forrest Gump*. A great scene is when Forrest and Lt. Dan were on the shrimp boat during the hurricane. Forrest was scared, but Lt. Dan was MAD! He was YELLING, "YOU WILL NOT SINK THIS BOAT!" And lo and behold, when the storm was over, that ship was still sailing! The same philosophy applies to you. When going through a storm (and you will go through one), stand up for yourself! Let them know that you will keep standing and will NOT sink! Life is full of storms, but your ship is strong and can withstand any weather thrown at it!

16. "May your life preach more loudly than your lips." –William Ellery Channing

Don't tell other people how wonderful, nice, thoughtful, kind, or awesome you are! Instead, let your actions speak for you! Or even better, be so BUSY doing what you claim that others are happy to do the talking for you!

17. "Don't stress about the closed doors behind you. New doors are opening if you keep moving forward." –Unknown

What if a basketball player dwelled on his last missed jump shot? Or a baseball player worried over the strikeout he had a couple weeks ago? What good would it be for a Broadway actor to remain upset about lines he forgot during a play 2 years ago? In each case, dwelling on the past miscues does NOTHING for them. Their best bet is to put it in their past and MOVE ON. It's the same with you. What's in the past is in the past. Dwelling on past mistakes will wear you out and wear you down!

18. "The will to win, the desire to succeed, the urge to reach your full potential...these are the keys that will unlock the door to personal excellence." –Confucius

Do you have the keys to reach your full potential? There's only one set. No duplicates, and YOU are the sole owner! If you have them, do you know how to use them? If you don't have them, find them! No one else can use YOUR keys!

19. "Be thankful you are still breathing. Someone out there just took their last breath." –Unknown
If you're reading this, you still have a chance. You still have a chance to change. If you're reading this, that means you WANT to make changes and you're either looking for inspiration or guidance. The fact that you CAN read this is all the inspiration and guidance you need! Don't waste your time dealing with people who complain ALL THE TIME, or with people who have no goals, dreams or morals. TODAY is your day to better yourself, as tomorrow is not guaranteed! Make today a great day!

20. "In order to bring me down you have to reach me." –Unknown
People will do to you what you let them! In other words, there are people out there who will take advantage of you and/or put you down, simply because you let them! Don't give people the opportunity to steal your joy, take advantage of you, or hurt you physically, mentally, or financially. You are on another level, and they only WISH they were where you are!

21. "Small minds can't comprehend big spirits. To be great you have to be willing to be mocked, hated, and misunderstood. STAY STRONG!" –Unknown
You are unique and wonderfully made! There's no one like you! With that said, don't be afraid to let your individuality show! Not everyone will see your vision, understand your point of view, or even agree with you, but do NOT let that stop you! EVERYONE who did something worthwhile had someone who TRIED to tell them it wasn't worth it or possible. Don't let someone else's opinion keep you from being the best you can be!

22. "When your past calls, don't answer. It has nothing new to say." –Unknown
Reminiscing over bad experiences does NOTHING for your present or future. Leave the past in the past. Whether it's a memory or person, if it was a bad experience, leave it where it was and don't look back!

23. "Ego says, 'Once everything falls into place I will have peace.' Spirit says, 'Once I find peace everything will fall into place.'" -Marianne Williamson

You will never be happy until you find peace within. No amount of money or material possessions can give you true happiness. Don't rely on external factors to make you happy, or wait to achieve a certain level in life. Be happy NOW, and when you get those material things, it'll be that much sweeter!

24. "I'd rather have a life of 'oh wells' than a life of 'what ifs.'" –Unknown

There's no telling how different your life would be if you try! Don't look back and wonder about what could've been. Do everything you always wanted to do NOW while you have time. There's nothing worse than wishing you would've at least TRIED!

25. "Anger, resentment, and jealousy doesn't change the heart of others, it only changes yours." –Shannon L. Alder

Is there anything worse than being angry or upset at someone, and they don't know or don't CARE that you're upset? YES, there IS something worse: You getting SICK from being angry or upset and they don't know or don't care! Or you becoming bitter and jaded, and taking those feelings and emotions out on people who had NOTHING to do with what upset you in the first place! Whatever is bothering you, you got to learn to LET IT GO for your health's sake. Leave that emotional TRASH behind!

26. "Faith is like WIFI. It's invisible, but has the power to connect you to what you need." –Unknown

Some people have faith in religion, some don't. Some have faith in their fellow man, some don't. Some have faith in their car starting or the bus coming on time, others don't.

Many of us will disagree on what to have faith in, but there's one thing we ALL should have UNSHAKEABLE, UNWAVERING faith in, and that's YOURSELF. Believe that YOU can do whatever you set your mind to! Oh sure, you can't see the path or how exactly it will get done, but that's where your faith comes in! Have faith that you will succeed, even when others don't!

**27. "Never put your key to happiness in someone else's pocket."
–Unknown**
Take CONTROL of your life! You are NOT a puppet on a string! Who makes the decisions for YOUR LIFE? You do, no one else does! Do NOT let someone else decide when YOU should be happy or successful. The time for you to take control is NOW! If you REALLY want something, go get it YOURSELF. Don't rely on someone else to give you what you want in this life!

28. "You don't have to go fast, you just have to go." –Unknown
I have a Bachelor's degree in Business Administration. It took 5 years and several summer school courses to get it. In 2010, I competed in the Florida Challenge Triathlon. I had mechanical issues on the 56 mile bike course and SEVERE leg cramps during the 13 mile "run" that forced me to WALK at least 9 of them. I finished the race in a little over 9 hours, DEAD LAST. But in both cases, I FINISHED.

My diploma is displayed proudly in my home. My finisher medal shines just as brightly as the first place finisher's. The concept of time is purely subjective. At the end of the day, the ONLY questions that matter are, Did you finish? Did you succeed? If the answers are yes, that's all you need! Whatever you're trying to do, do not give up! Just keep plugging away and you WILL get there!

29. "Every storm in your life is followed by a rainbow." –Unknown
Trials and tribulations are a part of life and we ALL will have our fair share of difficult times. No matter how nice you are, tough times are in your future too! While it may seem like the torture will NEVER end, stay strong! Things WILL get better! Don't overwhelm yourself. Take it one day at a time!

30. "Whatever you do, good or bad, people will always have something negative to say." –W. H. Auden
It's Time. It's time to understand that you CAN NOT PLEASE EVERYONE. It's time to start doing things YOU enjoy. It's time to stop worrying about what other people think. It's time for people to accept you for YOU. It's time to start living YOUR LIFE. Last but not least, it's time to do you!

**31. "Holding a grudge is letting someone live rent free in your head."
–Unknown**
Yes, they did you wrong. No, it's not fair. Yes, it hurts. Even with that
said, you have to learn to let it go. Holding on to those negative
emotions will prevent you from achieving the happiness you deserve!

When you have no one to motivate you or inspire you to keep going,
read some inspirational quotes, stories, and messages. They will give
you that extra energy to keep going when you didn't think you could.

PILLAR III

SPIRITUAL FITNESS

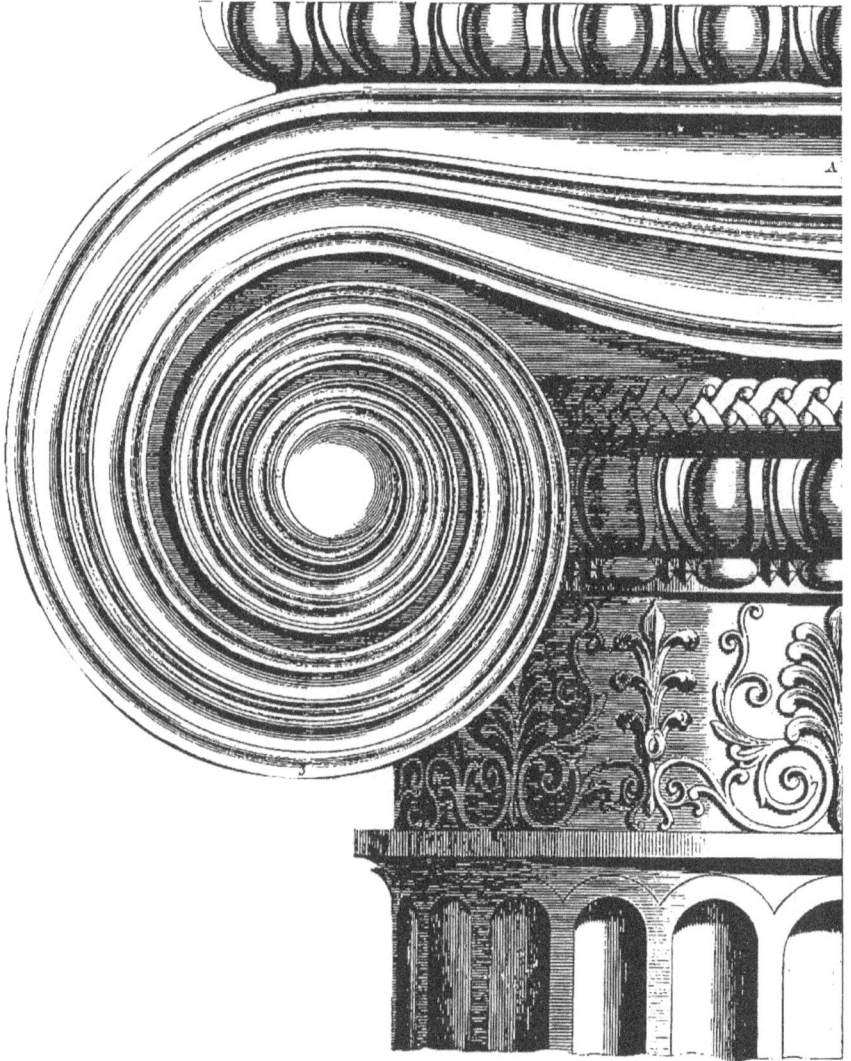

This section focuses on finding your inner peace, staying true to your convictions, and not bowing to peer pressure. Deep down we know the difference between right and wrong, but some will ignore these feelings and do things that can not only hurt themselves, but others as well. We will talk about resisting the urge to go against your inner voice, as well as attempting to right past wrongs. We'll also talk about material items and how the quest to obtain them can be detrimental to your physical, mental and spiritual health.

CHAPTER 19: RELIGION & SPIRITUALITY

I must stress again this book is about being the best you can be physically, mentally, and SPIRITUALLY.

This book is NOT to imply which religion a person should follow or which is the "best." The religion you follow is YOUR CHOICE and this book is NOT to tell you which religion is the one you should follow.

No matter what religion a person follows, they have a spiritual side, which is theirs and theirs only. Many people neglect this very important side of themselves, and THIS is what I want to focus on.

This is a self-help book where the principals can be used by anyone, regardless of their age, gender, ethnicity, sexual preference, or religious views. What we're referring to are morals and values that we ALL can relate to: qualities such as love, compassion, patience, tolerance, forgiveness, contentment, responsibility, harmony, and a concern for others.

If a person can understand the difference between the two, then we can begin to work on their Spiritual Fitness.

Out of the three sections of this book, the quest for Spiritual Fitness might be the most challenging for people to fully embrace—partly because it can be quite confusing. Many people believe that spirituality and religion are one and the same. For others they are separate, so it may depend on who you ask.

Let's look at the definition of spirituality:

According to Waaijman, the traditional meaning of spirituality is a process of re-formation, which *"aims to recover the original shape of man, the image of God. To accomplish this, the re-formation is oriented at a mold, which represents the original shape: in Judaism, the Torah; in Christianity, Christ; in Buddhism, Buddha; in the Islam, Muhammad."*

In modern times, the emphasis is on subjective experience. It may denote almost any kind of meaningful activity or blissful experience. It still denotes a process of transformation, but in a context separate from organized religious institutions, termed "spiritual but not religious," Houtman and Aupers suggest that modern spirituality is a blend of humanistic psychology, mystical and esoteric traditions and eastern religions.

On the other hand, religion is defined as a "belief in, or the worship of, a god or gods" or the "service and worship of God or the supernatural."

It's quite easy to see how a person can see them as the same, but according to the modern definition of spirituality, they can be separated.

This is important especially for those who don't consider themselves "religious" or follow certain religious beliefs. Even these individuals can tap into their spiritual side.

But before we really look at spirituality, let's look at some of the various religions around the world.

Judaism: The monotheistic religion of the Jews, having its ethical, ceremonial and legal foundation in the precepts of the Old Testament and in the teachings and commentaries of the rabbis as found chiefly in the Talmud.

Christianity: The religion based on the life and teachings of Jesus Christ. Christians believe that Jesus Christ is the Messiah, sent by God.

Islam: A religion, founded by Muhammad, whose members worship the one God of Jews and Christians (God is called Allah in Arabic) and follow the teachings of the Koran. Islam means "submission to the will of God". Adherents of Islam are called Muslims.

Baha'i: Monotheistic religion emphasizing the spiritual unity of all humankind. Three core principles establish a basis for Bahá'í teachings and doctrine: the unity of God, that there is only one God who is the source of all creation; the unity of religion, that all major religions have the same spiritual source and come from the same God; and the unity of humanity, that all humans have been created equal, and that diversity of race and culture are seen as worthy of appreciation and acceptance. According to the Bahá'í Faith's teachings, the human purpose is to learn to know and love God through such methods as prayer, reflection and being of service to humanity.

Hinduism: A religion of India that emphasizes freedom from the material world through purification of desires and elimination of personal identity. Hindu beliefs include reincarnation.

Taoism: A principal philosophy and system of religion of China based on the teachings of Lao-tzu in the sixth century B.C. and on subsequent revelations. It advocates preserving and restoring the Tao in the body and the cosmos.

Buddhism: A nontheistic religion that encompasses a variety of traditions, beliefs and practices largely based on teachings attributed to Siddhartha Gautama, who is commonly known as the Buddha, meaning "the awakened one."

Sikhism: A monotheistic religion founded during the 15th century in the Punjab region of the Indian subcontinent, by Guru Nanakand continued to progress through the ten successive Sikh gurus (the eleventh and last guru being the holy scripture Guru Granth Sahib. "The central teaching in Sikhism is the belief in the concept of the oneness of God." Sikhism considers spiritual life and secular life to be intertwined.

Scientology: Scientology is the study and handling of the spirit in relationship to itself, others and all of life.

Wicca: A religion influenced by pre-Christian beliefs and practices of western Europe that affirms the existence of supernatural power (as magic) and of both male and female deities who inhere in nature and that emphasizes ritual observance of seasonal and life cycles

Kabbalah: Ancient Jewish tradition which teaches the deepest insights into the essence of God, His interaction with the world, and the purpose of Creation. Kabbalah teaches the essential Jewish cosmology, integral to all other Torah disciplines. Sometimes called the "Inner Torah" or the "Wisdom of Truth", it offers a comprehensive structure and plan for the universe, as well as a detailed understanding of the particulars of our lives.

As of this writing, there are roughly 4,200 religions that are being actively practiced around the world according to estimates. This is just a small sample.

Other religions practiced around the world include the following:

Rodnoveri
Celtic pagan
Heathenism
Semitic pagan
Kemetism
Hellenismos
Roman pagan
Palo, Vodou
Servants of the Light
Sufism

"Worldwide, more than eight in ten people identify with a religious group," says a new comprehensive demographic study of more than 230 countries and territories conducted by the Pew Research Center's Forum on Religion & Public Life.

"There are 5.8 billion religiously affiliated adults and children around the globe, representing 84 percent of the 2010 world population of 6.9

billion," the analysis states.

Listed here is a rough approximation of 10 religions ranked by the number of members:

Rank	Religion	Members	Percentage
1.	Christianity	2.1 billion	33.0%
2.	Islam	1.3 billion	20.1
3.	Hinduism	851 million	13.3
4.	Buddhism	375 million	5.9
5.	Sikhism	25 million	0.4
6.	Judaism	15 million	0.2
7.	Baha'ism	7.5 million	0.1
8.	Confucianism	6.4 million	0.1
9.	Jainism	4.5 million	0.1
10.	Shintoism	2.8 million	0.0

Each religion has their own set of beliefs and principals, and people will gravitate towards a particular religion in a variety of ways.

Some people will study different religions and choose one they prefer after much thought and consideration. Others are literally born into it and practice a certain religion because their parents are followers and that's the primary religion in their region.

Some have a life changing event and turn to religion for strength and guidance.

Religion also gives members of the same faith (and other like-minded individuals) a way to worship and fellowship together: churches, temples, mosques, synagogues, and others are examples of where they would meet and have worship services.

These places of worship are held in high esteem: Under International Humanitarian Law and the Geneva Conventions, religious buildings are offered special protection, similar to the protection guaranteed hospitals displaying the Red Cross or Red Crescent. These international laws of war bar firing upon or from any religious building.

Politics and religion are two topics that people tend to avoid because people can get VERY passionate about their beliefs! Whatever religion a person follows, they might be likely to believe their religion is THE religion and the ONLY religion a person should follow.

It is such a passionate topic that people will get into heated discussions about their beliefs. Friendships and even family ties can be strained over religious differences. Over the course of history, wars have been fought with religious beliefs being a strong factor.

The ongoing Israeli–Palestinian conflict can be viewed as an ethnic conflict, yet elements on both sides view it as a religious war as well.

Other examples of religious conflict consist of:

-The Lebanese Civil War, between Christians and Sunni Shiite (1975-1990)

-The Second Sudanese Civil War between Islam and Christian (1983-2005)

-The Crusades in the 13th century were military campaigns sanctioned by the Latin Roman Catholic Church during the High Middle Ages and Late Middle Ages.

-The war in Bosnia-Herzegovina was among three faith groups, (Muslim, Roman Catholic, and Serbian Orthodox). (1992-1995)

There are many others, but the point I'm trying to make is how passionate people can be when it comes to their religious beliefs.

The ideals and principals of most religions are written down and are to be studied by their followers. The Torah, Koran, and Holy Bible are examples of such writings and have been around for centuries with little or no changes. The writings are the same now as they were when they were first written.

There are many books written on how to swim, run a marathon, shoot a basketball, or throw a football. There are also books on how to drive a car, bake a cake, or even put up a ceiling fan. That's all well and good, but until you get out there and actively use what you read, you'll never master the skill. You have to put in the time and energy to become good at that endeavor.

It's the same with tapping into your spiritual side. You can read about it all you want, but it's up to you to tap into your own spirituality and apply it to your everyday life. We all don't have the same patience, temperament, or life experiences that mold and shape us. It's because of these differences why books are good; but, they can't do it all for everyone. For the sake of this book, we will move forward with the belief that a person's spiritual side is theirs and theirs alone, and tapping into that spiritual side is something they must do alone, and is key when trying to be the best person you can be.

CHAPTER 20: THE QUEST FOR INNER PEACE

Spiritual Fitness starts from within, and inner peace is a must-have.

Inner peace (or peace of mind) refers to a state of being mentally and spiritually at ease, with enough knowledge and understanding to keep oneself strong in the face of discord or stress.

Having inner peace also means staying calm during difficult times and living stress-free. It may not be realistic to live stress-free 100% of the time, so the goal is to be stress-free the majority of the time.

This is extremely difficult to do for many people. Stress is everywhere and can eventually wear a person down. Stress can come in many forms:

Job pressures
Financial woes
Family issues (children, spouse, etc.)
Illness
Etc.

The key with inner peace is knowing that things out of your control will happen, both good and bad. Oftentimes, these events will happen unexpectedly and without warning. It's important to have that inner peace so when things DO happen (and they will) you can withstand and endure.

"We can never obtain peace in the outer world until we make inner peace with ourselves." –Dalai Lama

At its core, inner peace is learning to "let it go." Holding onto negative memories or constantly having negative thoughts will ensure that you never obtain the spiritual fitness that you deserve.

It will also ensure you can't fully enjoy life and live it to the fullest.

It's important to note that we ALL have fears. We all have doubts. We've all worried or been anxious about something in our lives. These feelings are normal, so this is not to say there is something wrong with you for feeling this way. Quite the contrary.

However, if a person does NOT have inner peace and know how to apply it, these negative feelings (and similar ones) could be triggered anytime someone or some THING upsets them. The trigger could be big or small. It doesn't matter as the end result of them being upset is the same.

It's very difficult to be happy and enjoy life if you're always worried or upset about something. Do you seek inner peace? If so, it's important to have use and apply these concepts as often as needed.

Having inner peace means **letting go of your fears.** Many times, we fear something that hasn't occurred yet. Our imaginations are running wild, looking at the worst case scenario. That does you no good and will guarantee you'll never have peace.

Closure: Some of us hold on to anger, bitterness, and resentment over things that have happened in our past. Sometimes those events happened YEARS ago.

I held onto the anger of my mother's passing for YEARS, and that prevented me from starting the healing process. When I was finally able to release my anger, I could start to have closure and began to heal.

Doubts and anxiety go back to repeatedly thinking about future events and imagining the worst case scenario. Ask yourself: *What am I doubting? What am I afraid of?* Don't be afraid to face these issues. Be honest with yourself. These could very well be tied into physical and mental fitness also.

It's important to remember that if something doesn't work out, use it as a learning experience. It is NOT the end of the world if something doesn't go as planned!

A perfect example is this book: I have spent more than a year writing this book. Do I have doubts about its success? Yes. Do I fear that it will be trashed by critics? Absolutely. HOWEVER, that's pure speculation on my part. I have no idea what will happen, and if it doesn't do as well as I'd like, I can accept that. I have done my best, and that's all I can do.

If it doesn't work, I will regroup and move on. Oh well, I tried! Yes, I'll be disappointed, but I know I gave it my best shot, and that's all I can do. I have no regrets and stand by everything I have written. I am at PEACE with what happens.

That's MY inner peace.

Emotional baggage: Carrying around the emotions from previous relationships (business or personal) will not only wear you down, but they can prevent you from cultivating and creating healthy new relationships. In the financial industry we had a saying: *"Past performance does not guarantee future results."* Just because your ex treated you horribly does not mean the next person will. Stop carrying with you those negative memories, and most importantly, don't bring those feelings and emotions into your new relationship. The person you're involved with NOW has nothing to do with what happened to you before they met you.

This book is designed to tie all three aspects of fitness together, and show how all three can be used in unison. For example, having inner peace goes hand in hand with mental fitness. In both instances, removing any negative thoughts from your mind is of utmost importance. A person can't be mentally strong if they don't believe in themselves and are full of negative thoughts about themselves or their abilities.

On the other hand, inner peace CAN be achieved even if a person has negative thoughts about themselves. They are just resigned to the way things are. They don't believe they can succeed and have accepted this as fact. They've given up, in many cases without even trying. They are at peace with having nothing, doing nothing, and never succeeding.

This type of thinking is a direct contradiction to being the best you can be mentally. A mentally fit person would see a new challenge or opportunity and give it their best effort to make it work. They don't put limits on themselves and talk themselves out of something before even try it. They will give it 100%, and if it doesn't work, they are at peace with it because they tried.

This is the inner peace we want to achieve. I'm at peace with not being a successful financial advisor. Why? Because I can look back on that time in my life and know I truly gave it my best effort. It just wasn't meant to be. Just because I want it, doesn't mean it's supposed to happen. Life doesn't work that way. I wanted two kids, but I only have one. Life's twists and turns only provided me with one child. I'm at peace with that also.

Don't confuse having inner peace with giving up too easily. What good is inner peace if you don't even TRY to achieve a goal?

Being resigned to stay with a job that you feel doesn't pay you what you're worth or doesn't appreciate you is NOT inner peace.

Being okay with being single because your last relationship ended horribly is not the inner peace we are striving for.

Would you be at peace with not being able to ride a bike because you fell off one time? After you dusted yourself off, would you get upset and say, "It's too hard," and that's it? Never to try again?

Technically, you could be at peace with your decision, but was it a wise decision? Is it possible you gave up too soon?

This is where mental fitness comes into play. This is where you tell yourself I will KEEP TRYING, and after I've tried over and over and over again and I STILL can't ride this bike, THEN I'll be at peace.

Inner peace is crucial, but don't sell yourself short. Make an effort to be the best you can possibly be. Make a serious effort to succeed, then let the cards fall where they may.

When the results come, live with them and learn from them.

That's the inner peace we're striving for.

CHAPTER 21: HAPPINESS COMES FROM WITHIN

As a whole, we are a materialistic society. Turn on the television and the actors and actresses have nice things and their lives are great.

Listen to some forms of music and their subject matter pertains to making money, driving nice cars or simply SPENDING money. The music videos give a strong visual on how money and the material items you can buy with it has made their lives that much better.

"They made it" is a common term for those who went from poor backgrounds to being successful. They are now living the "American Dream," and if you don't have a certain level of success, you aren't living *The Dream*. You're either not trying hard enough or you don't have what it takes to become a success.

Thanks to the internet and social media, this message (and others) are everywhere and may be practically impossible to get away from. As a result, many of our young people (and people in general) are raised with this thought: Get all the money you can, and anything less is a failure.

This isn't said outright, but it's subliminal. Young men are led to believe that in order to get the woman of their dreams they have to have cash: Pro athlete, entertainer, drug dealer, etc. are the professions that will get you the money (and the girl). It doesn't matter if you get it legally or illegally, as long as you have it is the message.

Some girls are taught to get the successful guy who can provide for them and the lifestyle they want for themselves and their family. No money? Don't waste her time.

I can do bad all by myself! is the motto for some women.

Now of course this doesn't apply to all people, but we all know someone who thinks along those lines.

Now let's be clear: There's NOTHING wrong with wanting nice things and being successful. There's nothing wrong with having money in the bank and having nice things. There's nothing wrong with building a fortune and setting up your family and generations to come to live comfortably. If a person achieves a certain level of success, why not treat yourself to a nice car, house, or other fancy items?

I don't think there's anything wrong with it, not at all. The problem is when people become so obsessed with getting money that they do almost anything to get it, or will delay their happiness until they DO get it.

We will talk more about people doing almost anything for money in an upcoming section, but for now, let's look at those who wait on getting nice things to be happy or feel like they're a failure because they DON'T have money.

In order to get anything of value, sacrifice is in order. You must be driven and focused on long-term goals. You must be patient and see what you want as clearly as the words you're now reading.

When your friends are out partying, you'll be home studying or hard at work. You'll go to sleep early because you have to get up at 5am to get things accomplished.

You're on a mission, and NOTHING will stop you from getting what you want, and that includes a seven-figure bank account.

Because right now, you're not happy. You hate where you live, and your car doesn't have A/C and needs a paint job. You barely have food in the fridge and all your bills are overdue. Life is a struggle right now and you're NOT happy in your current situation. You're angry, sad and frustrated all at the same time.

Sounds familiar?

You won't rest until you get it, and when you do, THEN you can relax, be happy and have a good time. Then and only then can you ease up and enjoy everything that money can buy!

These types are highly ambitious and highly motivated. They know what they want and have the self-determination and drive to get it. Business owners, managers, salesmen, entrepreneurs, etc. They have the blueprint to success and are following it to the letter. Tell them they can't do something and they will work that much harder to prove you wrong. They don't need your help or support.

Then there are those who are trying to get rich via other methods. They may not have the drive, resources, or self-discipline to work as hard as those previously described, but their desire for money and living a lavish lifestyle is just as strong.

These types are attempting to get money in the best ways they know how: Playing the lottery, gambling, or partaking in illegal activities like selling drugs or stealing are just some of their methods.

No matter HOW they get the money, their motives are the same: they want more money to live better and to be happy.

Ironically, many of them DO have the work ethic to get what they want in a legal way, but choose the shady, unethical or illegal route instead. If they applied this same will and determination in a more positive and productive manner, they'd be successful beyond their wildest dreams. But that's another topic for another day...

Does money really make things better? Is money the answer?

Many believe it is. Many feel money is the key to happiness and the "good life," and life without it is downright depressing.

A reported study in the International Business Times in 2011, incorporating interviews with more than 89,000 people in 18 nations, revealed that 15% of people in high-income countries reported having been depressed, compared with 11% of those in low- or middle-income countries. Depression rates were highest in the United States and France, eclipsing poorer countries like Mexico.

Why are they depressed? There are literally hundreds of reasons why a person could be depressed, and we touched on some reasons in a previous section. But for now, we'll look at it from an economical point of view.

Having money IS a good thing. Having to worry about how you pay your rent or feeding your family is stressful. But at the same time, money is NOT the answer to all your problems or will guarantee happiness.

Being spiritually fit has NOTHING to do with your bank account or what tax bracket you're in.

The study said 15% of people in the wealthiest countries are depressed, but who are they exactly?

According to an Australian study, the young and rich are seeking help for anxiety and depression at twice the rate of their poorer peers. Their observations follow Columbia University research that found depression and anxiety occur at twice the national US average in the children of families with an annual income of more than $170,000.

The US research found affluent children showed high rates of alcohol and drug abuse, eating disorders and criminal activity such as stealing from their parents or peers. A theory behind the rate of anxiety and depression is the pressure high-achieving parents put on their children. In this case, the parents might be pushing their kids a little too hard to be the best they can be, and the expectations might be too much for them. Or the kids are simply rebelling and don't want to live the life that their parents want for them.

Whatever the reason, many believe depression should NOT be an issue for the wealthy, but it is. The parents are now having to deal with children who are having issues, thus putting a strain on the entire family. These conflicts about money and living a certain lifestyle can make it extremely difficult to attain peak spiritual fitness.

On the flip side, what isn't surprising is that according to a 2009 Gallup survey, the rate of depression is nearly twice as high for Americans making less than $24,000 a year than it is for those with annual incomes above $60,000.

And as described before, regardless if a person is rich or poor, these depressed individuals may be taking antidepressants or other drugs to feel better when in reality, the medicine is not getting to the root of the problem. It's time to put money in its place.

CHAPTER 22: MONEY IS NOT THE ANSWER

In order to survive in this society, you need money. Food costs money. Housing costs money. Want a cellphone or cable? You need money. You want to retire? A new pair of shoes? You need money.

Money is needed for practically everything. Even this book costs money. I didn't take the time to write it for more than a year for free!

I say all this to point out that we DO need money. It cost me time, effort, and money to get this book out to the masses. We ALL need money and to say or pretend we don't is not being realistic.

With that said, in terms of being spiritually fit, you don't NEED money to be the best you can be. You don't have to make a certain amount per year or be in a certain tax bracket.

The confusion comes about due to people's expectations. They feel they must attain a certain level of success or stature to be happy. If they don't reach it, they're not happy, and if a person isn't happy, how can they can be spiritually at peace?

How can a person be at peace when they planned on being a self-made millionaire by age 30, but instead they are forced to get a part time job to make ends meet at a shoe chain, making a little more than minimum wage? That "person" was me, and I wasn't at peace. At age 30, my career as a financial advisor wasn't going as well as I had hoped. I worked on commission and hadn't received a paycheck in four months. I was ashamed to be seen working there and in a near panic. Truth be told, I thought I was a FAILURE because I was nowhere NEAR my financial goals.

I was obsessed with what I didn't have, but failed to look at what I DID have.

A couple years before this I did my first triathlon. I didn't even have a CAR at that time. I rode my cheap mountain bike TO the race, rode it to my job AFTER the race to pick up my check, and rode my bike HOME to my 300 square foot apartment.

Funny how looking back it was one of the best days of my life! And as I reminisce, some of my happiest memories didn't cost much money:

Riding my mountain bike along Lake Michigan; packing a sandwich and chips for my lunch as a teenager; going swimming in my apartment complex with friends as a teenager; and taking my son to the park and watching him run around and play.

My college life at Illinois State University was the greatest time period in my life, and I was ALWAYS broke! We all were, but I don't really remember that part. I remember all the great friends I made and still keep in touch with to this day, 20 years later.

One event my wife and I still talk about to this day is when we had a picnic on the beach when we were dating. We bought ready-made sandwiches and took a board game and had a GREAT time. That trip cost us practically no money, and we talk about that more than our honeymoon, out-of-town trips and expensive dinner dates. If you look back on your life, you'll see that you have MANY great memories and fun times that did NOT cost much money, if any at all.

Think about it. Think about the times you were out with friends laughing and having a good time and you had no money in your pocket or bank account. Laughter is free. Genuine friends who like you for you are free.

It's these things that you can truly enjoy whether you have money or not, and they are the key to happiness and enjoying life. Even back then, money may have been an issue, but you still found a way to enjoy life. Is it possible you could've enjoyed it MORE if you allowed yourself to relax and not be so focused on your lack of funds?

Looking back on your past, what did worrying about money (or lack thereof) accomplish?

I remember when I FINALLY got a car I was able to travel farther to triathlons. Never mind the car was almost 20 years old, had no air conditioning, was rusted, and had no lock for the driver's door. At the time it was a tad embarrassing to drive it anywhere, let alone to races where some bike WHEELS cost more than my entire car! Ironically, I look back on those days with NOSTALGIA and pure happiness.

It's quite funny when I think about it: All those fancy cars and bikes out there, and here I come with an old Buick and a bike I bought at the pawn shop for $100!

In actuality, I'd like to relive those "broke" days just one more time...

And even though I have more money and material items now than I did back then, my happiness hasn't increased just because my bank account has. My happiness has increased because my MINDSET has changed.

I'm still not where I want to be in life financially or otherwise, but I'm still working towards that goal. That's all I can do. I just have to stay productive and focused on getting where I want to be. But until then, I will live my life and enjoy it to the fullest, as there's no guarantee I'll get the things that I feel I should have.

Just because I want something doesn't mean I'll get it. I have accepted this important FACT of life and will still enjoy it, in spite of. So even if I don't get all the fancy items that I want, I'm richer in many other ways that money can't buy, and I'm fully aware of how "wealthy" I really am.

I have my health. There is no price tag on clean arteries or being free of disease. There are plenty of wealthy people in the hospitals (and morgues). The simple fact that I woke up with a sound mind and body and can keep striving to be the best I can be is priceless.

The beach. One of my favorite things to do is go by the beach. It clears my mind and puts me in a good place. Walking on the sand and listening to the waves cost nothing, but makes me feel alive!

After thinking for YEARS that we couldn't have children, my wife and I were blessed with a beautiful baby boy. No amount of money can take the place of having a happy, healthy family.

As I said before, the majority of my memories do NOT Include money or needing a lot of it. Even when I worked at that shoe store and was living check-to-check, I have nothing but good memories of those days.

This is just a small sample of things I'm grateful for and don't take for granted. We all have similar things in our lives. Think back to happy times in your past. How many of those great memories didn't need much money? Instead of focusing on what we don't have, it's better to focus on what you DO have.

Make no mistake, I still like, want, and need money, but my happiness will NOT be dictated by my bank account. If you're like me, you want to live a certain LIFESTYLE, and that lifestyle will cost money. But it's important to remember that a nice lifestyle will NOT guarantee you happiness or inner peace.

It is very important to understand this FACT. There are people living the life you want RIGHT NOW who are unhappy. Think about that for a minute. Not all of them, but there are some. If a person does not believe this they will have a difficult time finding the peace they deserve.

It's also important to understand that just because you have or get money doesn't mean you will ALWAYS have money. The National Endowment for Financial Education cites research estimating that 70% of people who suddenly receive a large sum of money will lose it within a few years.

In another study, a paper published in 2010 by researchers at Vanderbilt University, the University of Kentucky, and the University of Pittsburgh, authors looked at lottery winners and separated them into two groups: those who won sizable cash prizes (between $50,000 and $150,000) and those who won more modest prizes of $10,000 or less. They found that five years after the fact, the big winners were the ones more likely to have filed for bankruptcy.

It's not just the lottery winners who lose it all. Countless athletes and entertainers who made millions have filed for bankruptcy: Larry King, Burt Reynolds, Kim Basinger, Toni Braxton, MC Hammer, Warren Sapp, Donald Trump, Elton John, and Mike Tyson have all filed for bankruptcy. Even Mark Twain and President Ulysses S Grant (yes, THAT Ulysses Grant on the $50.00 bill) filed for bankruptcy.

Even savvy business people aren't immune to losing it all: In 2009, Bloomberg reports that wealthy individuals' Chapter 11 filings increased 73% in the second quarter from the year before. These are individuals with at least $1,010,650 in secured debt and $336,900 in unsecured debt.

The bankruptcies were tied to the real estate crash that swept across the United States.

In 2013, there were a total of 1,170,324 bankruptcy filings in the United

States, with 1,132,772 of those coming from individuals. As you can see, getting money and keeping it are not guaranteed. You could very well become richer than in your wildest dreams, only to lose it all in a few short years.

Now you may say, "That'll never happen to me!" But I imagine the celebrities above said the same thing, as well as the 1.1 MILLION individuals who filed for bankruptcy in 2013.

It COULD happen to you, which is all the more reason to NOT hinge your happiness on the size of your bank account.

Learn to be happy NOW. Don't let your spiritual and mental fitness be dictated by something that could be taken from you in a blink of an eye in a bad investment deal, tax audits, bad loans, or simply because you spent more than you had!

You are MUCH MORE than your bank account. Money can come and go, but the things money can't buy such as your health, self-respect, TRUE friends, and waking up in the morning are what's most important.

If you want to be wealthy and successful, by all means go for it! I know I am! But never forget that you are still rich with or without a large bank account!

CHAPTER 23: SELLING YOUR SOUL: HOW MUCH IS IT WORTH?

How much are you willing to do to be successful as discussed in the previous section? Don't lose your dignity or self-respect in pursuit of your goals and aspirations.

Your soul is priceless. There's no price tag that can be put on it and there's nothing on this earth that compares in value. Your soul is what makes you unique. It is that inner voice inside of you that tells you right from wrong and keeps you on the right path.

Your soul tells you when YOU'RE doing someone or something wrong, or when SOMEONE ELSE is doing you wrong. It's the inner voice that only you can hear, and even when it whispers, you can hear it loud and clear.

It's the voice that will wake you out of a deep sleep in the middle of the night to tell you what you're doing isn't right. It's the voice that tells you something about a situation you're in is "off." It may not tell you exactly

what it is, but it just knows something isn't right.
Some people choose to stop what they're doing and listen to this voice, while others pay no attention and move forward.

Listening to this voice is key to being spiritually fit and having inner peace. If the voice inside of you isn't happy, you won't have peace. The problem with this is when people choose to ignore their inner voice. They are so set on achieving a goal that they will do ANYTHING to get it.

Unfortunately, not everyone knows how dangerous this is. They don't understand how valuable their soul is and how important it is to your spiritual fitness. Instead, they act as if it's for sale and will sell it to the highest bidder or anyone who expresses interest.

Your soul is your everything, and without it, you're lost.

Our society puts a lot of emphasis on material items and being successful. It is strongly encouraged to be the best you can be. We are bombarded with images of what success is supposed to be, and if you don't have these material items or achieve a certain level of success, then you are a failure.

We are encouraged to live above our means and "keep up with the Joneses."

Turn on the television and you're bombarded with commercials of fancy items that you MUST have. Products that will make you happy and feel complete. Then there are stories and images of people who are doing better than you in life and having a great time doing it.

They're living their dream life, having a BLAST, while you sit in front of the TV watching them live that life.

The subliminal message is you're boring and you're missing out on all the fun. Everyone else is doing better than you and you're a loser.

We're taught to be ambitious, and that climbing the corporate ladder and being the best of the best is encouraged. "Win at all cost" is the mantra. Coming in 2nd place is considered "first loser."

Please understand there is NOTHING wrong with being the best you can be. We ALL should strive to achieve greatness in some aspect of our lives. That's the premise of this book: to be the best YOU can be physically, mentally and spiritually.

A person should always try to improve themselves because a person who becomes complacent can become stagnant and not grow. The world could literally go right past them and leave them in the past.

But there's a fine line with being the best you can be and winning at all costs. Some of us will get caught up in the media's portrayal of what success is, and far too many people are willing to cross the line to get that success:

In school, some students will cheat on tests to get good grades instead of getting good grades on their own merits. At their places of employment, some individuals will lie, backstab, and sleep their way to the top. In sports, some athletes will take illegal performance enhancing drugs to win or get an edge on their competition. In politics (and other areas of life), individuals will discredit others and slander their names just to make themselves look better and gain popularity.

These achievements are all built on lies and deceit, and those who have done any of the above know deep down that this is wrong. Now whether they care or not is one thing, but they do know deep down that this is wrong.

A person who builds their fortune or success in this manner has built it on a weak foundation that can crumble the instant someone decides to take it from them.

Pro athletes Lance Armstrong, Mayor Kwame Brown, Penn State football coach Jerry Sandusky, track star Ben Johnson, President Richard Nixon, stock trader Bernie Madoff, and many others have all been accused of scandals that drastically hurt their reputations and careers.

Not only did many of these individuals face jail time, but they were fined and condemned by the public at large. Once scandals like these and others similar have been exposed, it's very difficult to salvage your character or reputation.

All it takes is one angry person to alert the public about the wrongs they have committed and everything they worked so "hard" to build can crumble in an instant.

How many sleepless nights can a person have because they are worried they will be exposed? How paranoid will they be not knowing who their real friends are because they wronged so many people over the years? How difficult would it be to trust people, thinking they will be used the same way they used others?

This is not the way to live. There's no happiness in this type of life.

That inner voice is calling out to them, and no matter how hard they try, they can't silence it. No amount of drugs, alcohol, or other addictive vice will keep it quiet. Once they sober up, the voice returns. Over and over they will try to drown out the voice, only to have it return again and again.

No matter how "busy" they try to stay, sooner or later they will take a moment to rest, and when they do, that voice roll start talking to them (again).

It's enough to drive someone crazy with guilt, stress, anxiety, and worry.

With all these burdens and thoughts in a person's mind, the chances of having inner peace are very slim.

Now think about this for a minute: There are people who have sleepless nights, are abusing drugs or alcohol, have stress related illnesses, or other ailments due to their inner voice telling them they are doing wrong. After years and years of inner turmoil, their body is starting to wear down.

Not only is their spiritual fitness being affected, but their mental and physical fitness are now being compromised as well. A person who can't sleep may start taking sleeping pills. Another might get high blood pressure due to stress and start taking medications to manage it. A person who's trying to avoid their demons may abuse alcohol or illegal drugs, and may be doing severe damage to their liver and other vital organs.

As you can see, it's important to work on ALL aspects of your fitness as they are all intertwined. Society tends to look at just one aspect of a person's health, but our health can be affected by a variety of things, and it's important for a person to understand this.

If you have an ulcer, look into WHY you have an ulcer. Is it because you're been eating the wrong foods? Why are you eating those foods? Are they comfort foods? If so, why do you need comfort foods? Why do you need food to "comfort" you?

Do you eat certain foods when you're angry, sad, or depressed? What's causing these emotions?

Your doctor will NOT ask these questions. That's not their job. It's yours.

It's very possible your physical ailment (like an ulcer) is actually caused by inner demons that you've had for YEARS. Demons you have yet to acknowledge or deal with head on that are now eating you up inside. Literally.

If you want peace, you must face what's causing you anguish.

The time is NOW.

But there are other ways people sell their soul. There are those who will lie, cheat and steal their way to the top with no regard to those they hurt in their quest for success.

Not everyone is like this (of course), but we all know an individual (or two) who have done something as described above.

It may not happen immediately, but eventually, their conscience will start to eat at them. They'll start to reflect on their life and think about all the people they hurt or took advantage of on their way to the top. They'll look at their accomplishments and they'll start to feel hollow.

Who can they celebrate their success with? People who, if they knew the truth, wouldn't approve of their methods? Or people who appear to be happy but are secretly trying to take their spot the first chance they get?

They may not say it outwardly, but their inner voice will tell them that they were wrong and they didn't earn it the right way.

As I said before, there are those who have suppressed this inner voice, and for these individuals, they are a lost cause. They feel what they are doing is okay and no one can tell them otherwise, even though it is clearly wrong.

But for others, that inner voice will start to get louder and louder to the point where they have no choice but to start listening to it. It starts to eat at them and they become consumed with guilt.

Once this happens, the only way to have inner peace is to attempt to come clean or right the wrongs they have done.

Some people are willing to face these demons, while others try their best to suppress them.

An important aspect of being spiritually fit is being true to yourself. If you want to achieve the spiritual fitness that you truly deserve, it's important to be true to yourself from the beginning.

Resist the urge to demean and disrespect yourself (and others) to get ahead.

If you have to do all that, is it really worth it? Is that promotion really worth you posturing and playing up to your boss so much that you lose your identity and do start to do things you would normally disagree with?

How frustrating would it be to get laid off or fired after sucking up to the boss? After working so hard to kiss up, he STILL lets you go.

Is being part of the "in crowd" so important that you feel it necessary to smoke, drink, steal, join a gang, wear sagging pants, bully others, or disrespect women to be accepted?

Is it worth jeopardizing your future to not study in school to impress those who clearly have no goals, morals, and values? Is their acceptance and approval that important? Is that man so important to you that you

MUST sleep with the guy you just met, when you know deep down you're not ready?

When you do things like this (and others), you're no longer true to yourself. You're becoming someone else that in time you won't even recognize. Not only that, you're losing control of yourself and becoming someone else's puppet. THEY hold the strings and you are at their whim. You KNOW deep down these things you're doing are wrong, but you keep doing them for whatever reason.

You're slowly selling your soul to the highest bidder. Your soul is NOT for sale! Do NOT bow down to pressure to do things you KNOW aren't right!

Do NOT let the lure of a lavish life obtained in the wrong way compromise who you really are! There's no law saying you can't be successful by staying true to yourself!

If you feel compelled to do things in ways you disagree with and know they aren't right, find another way that goes with YOUR values and beliefs!

If your peers are forcing you to take drugs, it's time to find new friends because they are NOT your friends! A real friend would NOT force their friends to do something they don't want to do. Real friends accept you for who you are!

If a man really cares and respects you, he will WAIT for you to be ready for intimacy.

Your inner voice will keep you out of a lot of bad situations if you allow yourself to listen. That same voice will also tell you the good people to have in your life and who to avoid.

Do NOT be afraid to remove people from your life who clash with that voice. It may be difficult and you may experience resistance, but this is YOUR health we're talking about. No matter what you do, someone won't be happy with your actions but there is one person who MUST be happy, and that person is YOU.

LIVING WITH REGRET AND GUILT

As discussed in the previous section, doing things you know deep down are wrong can be very harmful to you spiritually, as well as physically and mentally over time. The effects may not be immediate, but as people reflect on their lives they may see the error in their ways and feel a sense of regret.

Regret and guilt are some of the hardest things to live with because you can't go back in time and redo your wrongs.

For the purpose of this book, regret is wishing you didn't do the things you did. Guilt is feeling bad for your actions and the damage they caused.

In both instances, once it's done, it's done. It's especially difficult when you have changed from the person you once were and don't condone your previous actions. As you reflect on your past transgressions, that inner voice may not only be talking to you, it may be SCOLDING you asking HOW could you had been so heartless and careless.

Some forms of regret and guilt can really hurt:
- The prisons are full of people who regret their past crimes.

- Individuals who took advantage of the elderly

- Those who bullied their peers

- Parents who abandoned or mistreated their children

- Individuals who are now alone because they were mean to their loved ones and/or took them for granted

- Murderers

- Drug dealers who destroyed their community

It's very possible that a person has changed and wouldn't do what they did before, but their past still torments them. Twenty years later, they can see the pain they caused as if were yesterday. Try as they might, they just can't shake these feelings.

As a result of their past, they aren't as fit spiritually as they could be. They can't go back and change anything, but they must do something in order to move forward.

These feelings are similar to carrying a 50 pound backpack and trying to pretend it's not there. It will weigh you down, and unless something is done to remove it, you won't be able to move through life as efficiently as you should. But once the backpack is taken off, a huge sense of relief will be felt and a person can move forward with their life guilt- and regret-free.

No one can make a person confront these feelings. They have to do this on their own terms, when they are ready. It's similar to a person addicted to drugs: going to rehab may be the best thing for them, but it's not going to be as effective unless that person wants to be there.

"Confront" is the correct term here because these may be feelings or emotions a person has ignored or denied for years—feelings that could be quite painful to deal with. But it must be done.

Here are steps a person can take to begin the process:

Write down your answers to these questions. Putting it down on paper is a good way to get the feelings out in the open and to start the healing process.

1. **What did you do? Why did you do it?** If you were in the same situation would you react the same or differently? Why or why not?

2. **Acknowledge the feelings.** Don't be afraid to admit to yourself what you did and the fact that it was wrong. Be honest with yourself. Why do you feel the way you do? Why do you regret or feel guilty about the situation?

3. **If you could handle the situation differently, what would you do?** This is a crucial first step. Being honest and truthful with yourself is the foundation to being spiritually fit. But this is just the first step. It's not enough to acknowledge the feelings. For example, a person could write

down, "I need to lose 20 pounds," but if that's all they do, it's just a waste of paper.

Wanting to lose those 20 pounds is improving your physical fitness. Wanting to get rid of the feelings of guilt and regret are part of improving your spiritual fitness. In both examples it's time for action. In some instances, no amount of time or effort will make things totally right, but it will still help give a person a sense of closure. A person may think it's too late to make amends and that may be true in some cases, but not in all situations.

A sincere effort to make things better in spite of the situation being different now could be just as beneficial to a person's mental state. They'll never know if they don't at least make an effort.

Here are some ways a person can cope with guilt and regret:

1. Stop abusing your body to cope. Drinking, drug use (legal or illegal) may help you deal with things in the short-term, but not only does it damage your body, it keeps you "busy."

Exercise in extreme cases can be another form of abuse and a method of escape; a person who isn't a pro athlete who works out every day, hours and hours on end might be trying to run from something.

In each case, a person doesn't have time to deal with the issue. This may help a person cope, but it doesn't get to the root of the problem. Time to stop running (literally) and right the wrongs.

2. Reach out to the person who was hurt from your actions. This may be one of the hardest things a person does. The last thing we may want to do is talk to the person we hurt. But just like you need closure, they need closure too.

Talking to this person may be painful and may reopen old wounds, but to move forward this is required.

It may be impossible to undo the hurt you caused, but it's amazing how far a sincere, heartfelt apology can take a person. Ask yourself: If someone who hurt you in the past reached out to you unexpectedly and apologized for the hurt they caused, how would you feel?

There are several ways you could take it:

1. Sense of relief. They finally get it! They understand the hurt they caused and are trying to make amends. Immediately forgiven.

2. Rage. The old feelings could come back to the surface and you let them have it. You really let them know how much you hate them. In a strange way, you getting these feelings out could be therapeutic. You finally get to let them know how much they hurt you. It may help you move on as well.

3. Indifferent. That person could try talk to you, but you refuse to acknowledge them or even listen to what they have to say. They keep trying to talk to you, but you continually refuse. They eventually give up.

In each case, there's some sort of closure involved. In the first case, it's a win-win. Everyone is happy.

In the 2nd case, both individuals leave the situation with very strong and powerful emotions. The meeting may have done more harm than good initially, but over time, they may be glad they got those feelings out and now have a sense of closure. The victim let them know how they felt, and the person who caused all the trouble got what they deserved. Both can now move on.

In the 3rd case, the person who caused all the trouble made a sincere effort to make amends. That is all they can do. If their efforts to apologize were rebuked that's not their fault. Depending on the situation and the severity of the guilt and regret, they can continue to try to make amends. That other person may just need more time to come around. They may not be ready to talk or acknowledge THIER pain.

Some things can't be rushed. Just because one is ready doesn't mean the other person is also ready. If you feel it's worth it, keep reaching out to that person. The breakthrough might be near.
In each of these cases, a person is one step closer to getting the inner peace they so desire. The key is to take action! Don't sit back and wait

for the right time or hope the feelings go away. The sooner you act, the sooner you'll be able to become spiritually fit.

But what if the person you need to talk to isn't around? What if the very people you need to talk to are nowhere to be found? Then what?

Reaching out to the person you hurt or mistreated years ago is crucial to achieving peak spiritual fitness. It's very difficult being the best person you can be when you have to deal with your past.

We just talked about reaching out to the person directly to make amends, but what if they are unavailable? What if they died years ago or you don't know how to reach them?

While complete closure may be impossible, there are some things you can do to help get some form of closure:

Treat people as if they are the person you hurt. If you were a bully in the past, be the person who defends others against bullies. Treat everyone you come across with respect.

Give back. Find an organization that supports individuals who were affected by your behavior and contribute to their cause. Abused animals? Donate pet food. Mean to a homeless person? Volunteer at a homeless shelter. Not there for your kids? Teased someone because they didn't have a father? Become a Big Brother or Sister.

Be creative! Find different ways to help out.

If all else fails, donate money. Every organization out there is on a budget, and if it's a non-profit they are probably working on limited funds so any contribution could help.

Please note: Don't just "throw" your money at something yet keep your old ways. Give your money but make an effort to change your ways at the same time. Your soul is NOT for sale and neither is your conscious.

Giving your entire paycheck to an organization may help them keep the lights on, but it won't help you achieve that spiritual fitness if you're not sincere with your donation. Do NOT offer your soul a bribe! That goes against everything we are trying to achieve.

Educate others. Looking back on my life, I wish someone would've pulled me to the side and told me when I was doing wrong. Even if I didn't listen at that specific time, the seed would've been planted and hopefully I'd heed their advice sooner than later.

This is where you come in. If you see someone doing things you KNOW they'll end up regretting or feeling guilty about, talk to them. Mind you, don't talk AT them, talk TO them. Most of us (myself included) don't like being talked down to. Many times, we'll tune that person out.

But if a person talks to me like I'm a real person, I'm more apt to listen. Even if I don't agree, I'll give them the same respect they give me.

Tell them your story. Let them know how you actually ENJOYED what you were doing, or saw nothing wrong with it. They will probably relate because that's how they currently feel. But something happened that caused you to change your perspective and now you regret those decisions. Tell them about the fallout of your actions, and how you made a vow to yourself that if you saw someone following in your footsteps, you'd at least talk to them.

Sometimes people just need someone to talk to. They need someone they can talk to one-on-one, in confidence. Someone who will listen to them instead of preaching and doing all the talking. They need someone to tell the ramifications of their actions. Someone they can relate to and respect. That person is you!

This is especially true of our young people. Many think they have all the answers, or simply don't have a positive figure in their lives to keep them on the right path.

Many of us are so busy simply trying to survive that we aren't taking the time to talk to each other. We're so focused on our own lives that we don't see the turmoil and anguish that could possibly be prevented if we just take a moment to TALK to each other.

Sometimes it's all about planting seeds. People may not listen to you or heed your advice right now, but it may simmer in their minds like food in a crock pot. It'll take time for what you say to sink in and all you can do is hope it does before it's too late.

If one person does this it's great, but if we ALL take this approach then we'd be much better off.

Guilt and regret are very difficult things to deal with, but there are ways to cope with it. Find the way(s) that help you reach your peak spiritual fitness and in time the rest of your life will slowly fall into place. And if you can help others with their spiritual fitness as you work on yours you'll be even more fulfilled and inspired to be the best you can be!

CHAPTER 24: THE PURSUIT OF HAPPINESS

Being spiritually fit has many different components. So far we have discussed having inner peace and ways to achieve it. A large piece of that puzzle is happiness. It's very difficult to be spiritually fit if you're unhappy.

Fact of the matter is we ALL should be happy. Each and every one of us should wake up with a smile on our faces, ready to start a new day with excitement and something to look forward to.

Unfortunately, that's not the case. Many people wake up in bad moods, sad, dreading the day, or simply tired from a lack of sleep.

Why are people so unhappy? The reasons are endless: They dislike their jobs; they're worried about money; they're not happy with themselves; they're not happy with their current situation, etc. Feelings of loneliness or isolation, or a sense of helplessness could also be potential factors.

This is a very small sample of why people are unhappy. No matter the reason, being spiritually fit is practically impossible unless some changes are made. There is much research being done on how moods, such as happiness and sadness, affect the brain. However, for the sake of this book, we will keep it as simple as possible.

There is one important determinant to happiness and that's a person's brain chemistry.

The human brain is very complex. So complex that scientists believe we only use 10% of our full capacity. It's also noted that a person's feelings and actions can release more (or less) of certain chemicals in the brain. For example, when a person is happy or in good spirits, chemicals released in the brain in response to happiness include endorphins, dopamine, serotonin and oxytocin. A study conducted by University of North Carolina researchers found that hugs increase the "bonding" hormone oxytocin and decrease the risk of heart disease.

Scientists and doctors have been studying the human mind for centuries and are still learning new things about how it works. Here's a brief description of chemicals that are key in terms of being happy—spiritually fit:

Endorphins: A hormonal compound that is made by the body in response to pain or extreme physical exertion. Endorphins are similar in structure and effect to opiate drugs. They are responsible for the so-called runner's high, and the release of these essential compounds permits humans to endure childbirth, accidents, and strenuous everyday activities. Endorphins reduce the sensation of pain and affect emotions.

Dopamine: Dopamine is both a neurotransmitter and a neurohormone that is produced in several different areas of the brain. Dopamine has a part in many important functions in the brain, playing a role in cognition, punishment, motivation, attention, mood, sleep, voluntary movement, learning, and working memory.

The brain includes several distinct dopamine systems, one of which plays a major role in reward-motivated behavior. Most types of reward increase the level of dopamine in the brain, and a variety of addictive drugs increase dopamine neuronal activity.

Serotonin: A chemical produced by the brain that functions as a neurotransmitter. Low serotonin levels are associated with mood disorders, particularly depression.

Oxytocin: Released from the posterior pituitary gland located in the brain. It is also known as the "hormone of love." It is released by both men and women when being intimate, and during childbirth.

As you can see, each chemical plays a vital role in a person's health and well-being. On the flip side, a lack of some of these chemicals in the brain has a negative effect.

Serotonin and norepinephrine are the main chemicals responsible for depression. Studies have shown that low serotonin levels in the brain can lead to anxiety, irritability, and sleep disorders that are normally associated with depression. Similarly, reduced levels of norepinephrine, a chemical responsible for arousal and alertness can lead to fatigue and a general depressed mood.

Dopamine is another chemical in the brain that can cause depression in a few cases. Another fact about dopamine is that it is associated with addiction of alcohol and drugs, which can stimulate its production in the body.

For example, a study from the University of Adelaide in Australia shows addictive behaviors in adolescents and adults are influenced by low levels of the "love hormone" oxytocin during early childhood.

External influences over the oxytocin system of a developing child may include stress, trauma, severe infection, or early exposure to drugs. And although these influences may not affect hormone levels, oxytocin itself becomes less responsive.

It should also be noted that many studies have been conducted on the symptoms and diseases related to oxytocin deficiency including the following:

Menopause & Surgical Menopause
Prolonged Stressful Situations
Hypothyroidism

Depression (including post-partum depression)
CMV infection
Multiple Sclerosis
Fibromyalgia
Feelings of Loneliness
Anxiety Disorders
Certain forms of Schizophrenia
Autism

As said before, this is a very basic explanation of each of these chemicals that are released by the brain. Research is still being done to see if there is a link between low levels of oxytocin and the illnesses above. There are countless in depth studies that go into much more detail about the complexities of the mind and how these chemicals affect it. The point here is to understand how happiness and feeling good truly start from within, and that your quest for spiritual fitness could be affected by something you're unaware of.

We must look at the big picture. The imbalances in any of the above can wreak havoc on a person and make it that much more difficult to have happiness and inner peace. All this is important because a person may be unhappy or upset and have no idea why. They may not even know they have an imbalance. The smallest things may cause them to go into a fit of rage, sadness, or depression.

They may start to use drugs (illegal or prescription) to make them feel better, or focus on material items to make them happy or feel good. They may need a glass (or two) of wine or their favorite alcoholic beverage to relax or feel good.

Before taking a drug or having a drink to feel better, it's important to know WHY a person is unhappy or distressed in the first place. Many times, we want to treat the symptom but not look at the root cause of the problem. Being the best you can be physically, mentally and spiritually means knowing what makes YOU tick and being in tune with your own body.

Sometimes simply knowing what's wrong is a huge milestone and a big first step on the road to recovery.

ANTIDEPRESSANTS

For some, being happy is not as easy as it should be. As described in the previous section, there may be some issues they have to address on a chemical level before they can feel what true happiness Is.

Prolonged sadness (for whatever reason) can have serious effects on a person. Current Medical Diagnosis and Treatment reports that prolonged depression or sadness can induce changes to mental health, physical health, physical appearance, and personal relationships.

Being spiritually, mentally, and physically fit are all but impossible if a person is dealing with these issues. A person's mood can alter their brain's chemistry. The changes that take place as a result of depression can appear as forgetfulness, listlessness, lack of motivation, despair, and discouragement.

It's crucial that a person understands what's going in in their mind (literally) and makes an effort to seek treatment. The type of treatment a person chooses is very important. Our society has been taught to believe that the answer to every ailment and malady is in a pill.

According to a report released by the National Center for Health Statistics (NCHS) in 2011, the rate of antidepressant use in the U.S among teens and adults (people ages 12 and older) increased by almost 400% between 1988–1994 and 2005–2008.

One way some antidepressants work is by altering the balance of certain chemicals in your brain. Others work by blocking a receptor in the brain that absorbs the chemical serotonin.

The federal government's health statisticians figure that about one in every 10 Americans takes an antidepressant. And by their reckoning, antidepressants were the third most common prescription medication taken by Americans in 2005–2008.

Antidepressants are known to have many side effects. Not everyone will experience every known side effect, but they are likely to experience a few as described below.

Nausea
Increased appetite and weight gain
Loss of sexual desire and other sexual problems, such as erectile dysfunction and decreased orgasm
Fatigue and drowsiness
Insomnia
Dry mouth
Blurred vision
Constipation
Dizziness
Agitation
Irritability
Anxiety

If a person is taking antidepressants to feel better, how happy are they going to be if they have weight gain, sexual dysfunction, and/or insomnia issues?

How probable is it that a person who unknowingly has insomnia due to antidepressants takes a sleeping pill to help them sleep?

If you're currently taking prescription pills, you're not alone. More and more people are taking multiple prescription pills. According to the CDC, over the last 10 years, the percentage of Americans who took at least one prescription drug in the past month increased from 44% to 48%. The use of two or more drugs increased from 25% to 31%. The use of five or more drugs increased from 6% to 11%.

In 2007-2008, 1 out of every 5 children and 9 out of 10 older Americans reported using at least one prescription drug in the past month.

Each of these pills tend to have their own side effects, which could be harmful to a person's health. So again, the question is how spiritually fit can a person be if they are taking multiple pills every day? How spiritually fit can you be if you're using medicines that affect certain chemicals in your brain?

This section pertains to spiritual fitness, but a person's physical and mental fitness is directly affected as well from these medications. As I said in the introduction, many of us live our lives like a jigsaw puzzle and neglect to put all the pieces together. Things we do can (such as taking anti-depressants) have a ripple effect and affect other aspects of our lives.

At this point, a person may be thinking they should stop taking their antidepressants altogether. This is not wise as it's advised that a person should gradually stop taking their medications with the help of a physician.

There are many withdrawal symptoms a person could experience including the following:

Anxiety
Fatigue
Nightmares
Trouble sleeping
Depression and mood swings
Loss of coordination
Muscle spasms
Dizziness
Difficulty balancing
Nausea
Vomiting
Flu-like symptoms
Headache

Not everyone will experience these symptoms, but they may experience some of them. Other more serious side effects are suicidal thoughts, a relapse, or an imbalance in other medications you're taking.

It is strongly advised that any decrease in medication is done under a doctor's supervision!

Our society is taught to take a pill as the first, and in some cases, the

ONLY option. We shouldn't have to take a pill to be happy. We shouldn't have to endure uncomfortable side effects when taking a pill to be happy.

In some cases, prescribed medications are indeed necessary, but are they needed in all cases? No, they are not. Before a person takes medications, they should explore other natural options.

The next sections will explore natural, safer methods to use in your Pursuit of Happiness, as well as what foods to avoid.

THE DIET OF DEPRESSION

As a society, we are encouraged to see a doctor and take a prescription or over-the-counter medication at the onset of disease or sickness.

There are instances where taking medication is needed, and in no way does this book imply or suggest a person should NEVER take medicine. What I'm saying is many people in our society see medication as the first and ONLY choice, and this is a mistake.

Every day our bodies are bombarded with germs and fights off disease. A healthy immune system can fight off these invaders, but if that immune system is worn down and weakened over time, those germs that had no effect in the past will start to take their toll on you.

With that said, it's important to keep your immune system as strong as possible, and that means being mindful of the foods you eat.

It should be noted that there are studies that link a bad diet to depression. In a study published in the journal *Brain, Behavior, and Immunity*, for 12 years researchers tracked the diet habits and health outcomes of more than 43,000 women—none of whom had depression at the start of the study period. Here's what they found: Women who sipped soft drinks, ate fatty red meat, or consumed refined grains (like pasta, white bread, crackers, or chips) daily were 29 to 41% more likely to be diagnosed or treated for depression than those who stuck to a healthier diet.

It is believed that the following foods can trigger depression:

Alcohol: Alcohol affects the chemistry of the brain, increasing the risk of depression.

High fructose corn syrup: Fructose (and lactose) can react chemically with tryptophan—the amino acid precursor for our important happy chemical, serotonin. The sugars can degrade tryptophan so that there isn't as much available to be absorbed in the body.

High sodium intake: Excessive salt intake impacts both your electrolyte balance and your hormones. It can severely hinder the conduction of nerve impulses and induce symptoms like dizziness, muscle cramps and shakiness. You can also have impaired sensory response and feel disoriented and nauseous. Studies have shown that a high salt diet can often lead to higher stress levels and overeating, making you much more susceptible to depression, anxiety, and obesity.

Artificial sweeteners: There are many health problems linked to artificial sweeteners. Studies show the phenylalanine in aspartame dissociates from the ester bond and increases dopamine levels in your brain. This can lead to symptoms of depression because it distorts your serotonin/dopamine balance. It can also lead to migraine headaches and brain tumors through a similar mechanism.

Individuals who consume a diet high in artificially sweetened drinks are more likely to experience a decline in kidney function, according to a paper presented at the American Society of Nephrology's annual meeting in San Diego, California. It can also cause neurological problems, including anxiety, dizziness, spaced-out sensation, and depression.

The ingredients on this list include a large variety of the foods and beverages many of us eat on a daily basis: Chips, donuts, cookies, soda, candy, lunchmeat, pre-packaged processed foods, soda, beer, artificially flavored foods and drinks, fast food, etc.

Many of us know how these foods affect us physically, but aren't aware how they can affect us psychologically, which studies show in a very dramatic fashion.

So now, if you've been diagnosed with depression, the questions that need to be asked are the following:

Are you on anti-depressants?
Do you eat any of the above listed foods on a daily basis?
Has anyone suggested you change your diet?
How is your overall health? Overweight, diabetes, high blood pressure, etc.?
Are you taking any other medications?

If these foods are believed to play a part in depression, how much will those meds help if you're still eating them while taking those meds?

How can you begin to get better if you're still doing things (unknowingly) that may cause depression in the first place, which includes eating foods that may aggravate your condition? Again, these are questions you must ask yourself, and you must be ready to make changes in your life if you want to get better.

Another thing to consider are "comfort foods," which was discussed in a previous section. When many of us are stressed or under duress, we turn to food or alcohol to make us feel better. The problem here is many of the foods we are eating to make us feel better are actually making us feel worse.

The foods we eat make it extremely difficult to be physically, mentally, and spiritually fit, and if we're taking medicines like antidepressants on top of it, being the best we can be is impossible. Even if the depression isn't caused by the products listed above, eating them will make getting better that much harder.

Even if a person doesn't know what causes their depression, a good first step is to change their diet by eliminating the unhealthy foods and eating clean, natural foods. There's no guarantee this will cure a person's depression, but it's a step in the right direction!

EATING YOUR WAY TO HAPPINESS WITH HERBS

As said before, this book is not anti-medicine. There are times when taking medicine is critical. The problem is when people use medicine as their *first* and *only* choice. People abuse their bodies by eating too much junk food, not getting enough exercise, and living an unhealthy lifestyle that over time catches up with them. When they get sick, they turn to the doctor for help. What many don't understand is that the doctor isn't your first line of defense against disease and illness. It's the foods you eat.

In the previous section we touched on the link between food and depression. While some may not agree with this connection, it's not out of the realm of possibility. If foods can be a primary factor in weight gain and other physical issues such as high blood pressure, heart disease and high cholesterol, why can't it also affect you on a more psychological level?

A happy body is a healthy body. If we are to be happy, that means we are disease- and drug-free, and that includes being free of prescription drugs. The next sections will highlight some foods, herbs, and other natural remedies that could possibly help depression and other chemical imbalances.

Please note: If you are taking medications, please consult with your physician before changing your dosages.

DO NOT STOP TAKING YOUR MEDICINE IN LIEU OF THESE SUGGESTIONS.

Herbal remedies.

Herbal remedies have been used for 3,000 years, with recorded use by Egyptians and Babylonians. Herbs can be traced back to the beginning of Ayurveda science in India, with China using and specializing in the healing properties of herbs ever since their discovery. Herbs are still used in many cultures presently to cure diseases and promote a healthy body and mind.

Herbal teas have many benefits, but for now, we'll just focus on the mental health benefits:

Asian Ginseng is an herb that may be beneficial in restoring your hormone imbalance. It can be taken in pill form or added to teas and soups.

Ashwagandha is an herbal remedy that may be effective in treating hormone imbalance. According to the Memorial Sloan-Kettering Cancer Center, ashwagandha is a popular Ayurvedic herb used to help treat stress, fatigue, pain, and diabetes. This herb does not need to be cooked to be consumed, and there are no specific guidelines for cooking ashwagandha. This herb can be added to teas or sprinkled on oatmeal in powdered form.

Ginkgo biloba is well known as a mood enhancer. It increases blood flow to the brain and may help to regulate the brain's neurotransmitters. It is used primarily in teas.

Siberian ginseng also helps to regulate the neurotransmitters. It has also been known to provide more energy and aid in concentration. Typically, only a small amount is suggested for each serving, such as a pinch for use in teas or soups. Other names for this herb are Devil's Shrub, Eleuthero, Siberian Ginseng, Touch-Me-Not, and Wild Pepper.

Valerian is another highly regarded herbal remedy for depression. Specifically used to lessen anxiety, it is a big help in allowing you to get back into social interactions. The best way to prepare and drink valerian root tea is with warm water at about 85 degrees Fahrenheit.

Valerian root is considered safe, although allergic reactions are possible, according to the University of Maryland Medical Center. Large doses of valerian root tea may lead to headaches or drowsiness, so you shouldn't drink it if you are going to be driving or operating machinery.

Note: It is suggested to not use boiling water with most herbal teas because some of the phytochemicals are sensitive to heat and may be destroyed. It's also advised to steep all herbal infusions for at least 10 minutes, if not for 30 minutes, to ensure that all of the beneficial components are released from the plant and infuse the warm water.

Next to water, tea is the most popular beverage in the world. Substitute the sodas and artificially flavored drinks that are popular today with the herbal remedies listed above. Honey is a great natural sweetener that has antibacterial properties and also contains flavonoids and antioxidants, which help reduce the risk of some cancers and heart disease.

Some of you might be wondering how long you should try these herbal remedies before you start to reap the benefits. I can't answer that as each person is different, but what I will say is this should be a part of your life, FOREVER.

This is a lifestyle change. It's not like taking medicine for a couple weeks, you feel better, then resume your old ways. It doesn't work that way. You are changing your habits for the better. Forever.

Personally, I drink green tea 4-5 days a week, and have been doing so for several years. Sipping herbal tea throughout the day is an easy and simple way to strengthen your body and help you achieve the happiness and inner peace you deserve. However, not everyone likes tea or many of the herbs that can be used in tea. If you don't like tea, seek alternative ways to use these herbs. Use the herbs in powder form and sprinkle them over oatmeal, smoothies, or other foods. Seek out recipes and be creative. This is YOUR health we're talking about. Don't wait on someone else to tell you how to take care of yourself. Look for ways you can use these herbs in your daily life and your body will thank you!

FOODS FOR A HAPPIER, HEALTHIER YOU

As shown in previous sections, happiness truly starts from within. It is well documented that prolonged anxiety and depression can be linked to chemical imbalances in the brain.

Herbal remedies are great ways to help treat anxiety and frustration, but a person can only drink so much herbal tea!

It is important to note that many of the processed foods, alcohol, sodas, and artificial sweeteners we eat on a daily basis can affect the chemicals balances in the brain, which have the potential to trigger depression. On the flip side, there are foods believed to help restore the brain's chemical balances to a more normal state.

Many of the foods we eat when stressed or upset (comfort foods) may taste good, but actually they make us feel worse in the long run. (Some of the more popular comfort foods are cookies, cakes, ice cream, alcoholic beverages, and fast food. We touched on this in the Physical Fitness section, but again, these are all interconnected.)

The more anxious or depressed a person is, the more they may reach for that ice cream, cookies, or alcohol to relax them or make them feel better.

Eating these foods could have a domino effect, meaning the results of eating too much over time could be a contributing cause of depression and other ailments such as hangovers, gaining weight, elevated blood pressure, diabetes, and stomach problems such as ulcers, among others.

It's not hard to believe that having to deal with these (and other health issues) could be depressing for some.

Is it possible the person dealing with ulcers is depressed? How upset would you be if you were just diagnosed with diabetes and told you must give yourself shots for the rest of your life?

Remember: This section of the book is titled The Pursuit of Happiness. How difficult is it to be happy if you're sick? What if the foods you're eating and the lifestyle you're living are contributing to your unhappiness?

A person who is depressed might be lacking in certain nutrients and don't even know it. The body needs extra tender loving care and nutrients when in this state, but instead of eating nutritious foods that will help, they eat junk food that could make their situation worse.

Here's a list of some of the vitamins and nutrients that could be lacking in a person suffering from depression and the foods that could help them:

Vitamin C: Strawberries, oranges, kiwi, pineapple, cranberries, grapefruit, cherries, blackberries, mango, broccoli, celery, red cabbage, red peppers, watercress, tomato, pumpkin, artichokes, asparagus, Brussels sprouts, cucumber, leeks, potatoes, radishes, spinach

Vitamin B3/B6: Brown rice, oats, barley
Beef liver and kidneys, chicken, turkey, pork loin
Tuna, salmon, trout
Chick peas, sunflower seeds
Watercress, cabbage, peppers, potatoes, squash, mushrooms, broccoli.
Bananas (low quantities of B6)

Magnesium: Oatmeal, long grain rice, barley, wheat bran
Walnuts, pistachios, peanuts, almonds
Sunflower seeds, pumpkin seeds
Strawberries, blackberries, orange, raisins, bananas
Broccoli, sprouts, peppers, watercress, spinach

Tryptophan (essential amino acid): Almonds, pecans, peanuts, hazelnuts
Milk, cheddar, Swiss cheese
Sesame seeds, pumpkin seeds
Turkey, chicken
Soya beans, kidney beans
Bananas, figs, dates

Zinc: Mozzarella, cheddar
Kidney beans, chick peas, lentils
Chicken legs and thighs, turkey, lamb, pork, minced beef

Spinach, broccoli, asparagus
Kiwi, blackberries
Walnuts, almonds, cashews

Omega 3: Walnuts
Salmon, mackerel, fresh tuna, trout, shrimps

Selenium: Calves liver, turkey
Shrimps, cod, halibut, salmon, tuna
Mozzarella
Sunflower seeds
Spinach, mushrooms, garlic

Folic acid: Calves liver, turkey
Lentils, chick peas, kidney beans
Spinach, lettuce, asparagus, sprouts, parsley, broccoli, green beans
Walnuts, cashews, peanuts, hazelnuts
Tuna, salmon, cod

It's crucial you change your mind set when feeling stressed, anxious or depressed. Instead of reaching for that cookie or soda to feel better, try eating the foods listed above. Eating a healthy diet is key when battling depression.

Below are specific foods in more detail that are known to have calming effects and are good for the mind:

Blueberries: The vitamin C combined with the many other antioxidants contained in blueberries fight cortisol, which is the stress hormone.

Blueberries are rich in antioxidant polyphenols such as anthocyanin's, which have been researched for their protective properties, particularly against aging and oxidative stress. Also, the fiber in blueberries helps to control blood sugar levels, and high blood sugar often leads to stress and anxiety.

A handful of blueberries daily could work wonders over time. Try these tips to incorporate blueberries into your daily diet:
Add to a smoothies

Use as jelly or jam
Eat with other fruits such as strawberries for a snack
Use in cakes, pies, pancakes, and breads

Almonds: Almonds are rich in vitamins B2 and E. Both of these nutrients help bolster the immune system during times of stress. Vitamin E has been shown to fight the free radicals associated with stress, and in particular, those free radicals that cause heart disease.

Spinach: Spinach is rich in magnesium, which helps regulate cortisol levels and promote feelings of well-being. Chronically elevated cortisol levels can cause a variety of ailments including thyroid and metabolic dysfunction, cognitive decline, low serotonin levels, resulting in depression, irritability, anxiety, and carb cravings, to name a few.

Dark chocolate: Dark chocolate helps to release serotonin and relaxes the blood vessels of the cardiovascular system. Cocoa also contains monoamine oxidase inhibitors (MAO Inhibitors) which help improve our mood because they allow serotonin and dopamine to remain in the bloodstream longer and circulate in the brain without being broken down.

If you're suffering from depression, it's critical that you take a hard look at your diet. The foods you eat may play a major role in your illness and a change in the foods you eat may be just what you need.

These changes are lifestyle changes, meaning you can't eat these foods listed here for a couple weeks then go back to your old habits once you feel better. Eating healthy foods daily will get you that much closer to the happiness you deserve!

TAPPING INTO YOUR INNER HAPPINESS

Depression and anxiety affects millions of people worldwide. We are conditioned to seek medical treatment for relief and while it is needed in some cases, there may be things a person can do to relieve their depression and anxiety that don't require medication.

As you can see, there are many foods and herbs a person can use to help their symptoms, but the push is to go straight to the meds first for relief.

Many will take meds in hopes of getting better, but they don't try to get to the root of their depression or try to determine what's making them depressed in the first place. A person could very well take pills for years, but it's all in vain if they continue to do the things that are causing their depression or anxiety in the first place.

So, in addition to herbs and foods, here are some other things people can do to alleviate that stress and anxiety:

Get a hobby: What do you enjoy doing? Having a hobby will keep you preoccupied and keep your mind off your problems.

Read books, solve crossword puzzles, learn to play an instrument or learn a new language. Find something positive that will keep you mentally stimulated.

Exercise: Working out is a great way to relieve stress as well as get you in shape. The key here is to find something YOU enjoy, not what is trendy or the current "in" thing to do. Walking is a great way to relieve stress and boost your mood. Not your thing? Try rock climbing. Or Zumba. Or scuba diving.

Another great idea is to find an activity that you have to work to achieve: Train for a 5k, 10k or triathlon. Having something to look forward to and work toward will help give you a sense of purpose and accomplishment.

Join a group or organization: Many depressed people feel a tremendous sense of loneliness. To help overcome this feeling, join an organization with individuals who share some of your likes and interests. Join a fraternity or sorority, book club, ethnic groups, religious or spiritual groups, runners groups, singles groups, etc. There is a group out there that would like to have you as a member. Find it and make new friends!

Get a pet: Studies show that pets can be relaxing and distract us from the things that may be bothering us. They also give unconditional love. Not sure what to get or don't think you have the time for a pet? Get a fish tank. Studies indicate that merely watching fish lowers blood pressure and muscle tension in people about to undergo oral surgery.

Breathe deeply: Stress and tension contribute to shallow breathing. Shallow breathing is also known medically as hypopnea, may result in hypoventilation, which could cause a buildup of carbon dioxide in an individual's body, a symptom known as hypercapnia.

By deepening your breath and keeping the rhythm consistent, you increase the amount of oxygen that is reaching your lungs, blood, organs, and cells. This oxygen, of course, is vital for your physiological systems to operate properly. Deep breathing also relaxes your body and mind so that you can examine your negative thoughts and replace them with positive ones.

Focus on relaxing and breathing slowly and deeply every time you think about it. This simple move could possibly relax you and put you in a better state of mind.

Change your mindset: It's important to understand there are many things out of our control, and worrying about them or trying to analyze them is not good for your health.

It's important to learn how to let things go and not let the unknown or things out of your control consume you. (This is talked about more in the Mental Fitness section of the book.)

Start laughing: A good laugh helps you mentally and physically. Watch funny movies. Read humorous books and seek out things and people that make you laugh. According to the Mayo Clinic, laughter has many benefits, including soothing tension. Laughter can also stimulate circulation and aid muscle relaxation, both of which help reduce some of the physical symptoms of stress.

Laughter may ease pain by causing the body to produce its own natural painkillers. Laughter may also break the pain-spasm cycle common to some muscle disorders.

Many people experience depression, sometimes due to chronic illnesses. Laughter can help lessen your depression and anxiety and make you feel happier.

This is just a small sample of things a person can do to help alleviate their depression. However, for this to be effective they all must be done together. Get to know your body and what makes it tick.

Don't just get a fish tank, yet keep your diet the same and expect everything to be okay. The key is to work on ALL of your aspects of your life at the same time. Start putting your jigsaw puzzle together slowly but surely, one piece at a time. It will take time for these suggestions to help, but the key is to get started.

Our bodies are very intricate and have the ability to heal and strengthen themselves if we give it the appropriate tools!

Medication should not be your first option. Do everything you can to help yourself before seeking meds. If these methods don't seem to be working, then seek medical advice. You may have issues that require medical attention.

We ALL deserve to be happy. Don't let another day go by where you are denied this right. Start your pursuit of happiness today!

CLOSING REMARKS

This book isn't designed to tell you what to do. It's to let you know you have all the tools to succeed inside you. The problem is we don't use all our tools together in harmony.

If you were building a house, you wouldn't use just a hammer, a saw, or a drill. If you only brought a socket wrench to build a house, you'd be laughed at and told you didn't know what you were doing.

It's the same philosophy with you and your personal growth. They say your body is a temple, and that means you need a variety of tools to build a temple that's fundamentally sound and has a strong foundation. The tools all work together and could be used at any time.

Since this is YOUR temple, and YOU are the architect, it's up to you to decide when you'll need the appropriate tools. It's not "if" you'll need them, it's "when."

You will need varying degrees of mental, physical and spiritual strength many times in your life. It's up to you to channel these various strengths and use them as needed. It's also very possible that something you thought took physical strength ONLY to accomplish also needs a good dose of mental and spiritual strength as well.

I believe that deep down, we all know this. When we lay awake in bed at 2 am, staring at the ceiling, these thoughts (or something very similar) may creep into our minds. They make sense at the time, but they are dismissed when we get up hours later and begin our hectic days.

Unfortunately, some of us don't know how to tap into this power because it's not talked about by those close to them or it isn't seen on a daily basis. Or we're so busy just trying to survive day-to-day that we don't think about it.

This book was written out of anger and frustration. Instead of taking my negative feelings and energy out on others, I decided to take them out via pen and pad.

Exercise is a great stress reliever for me, but this was different. This book is the result of conversations and things I've seen and experienced over the years.

I know too many people who are just trying to survive: Working 8-10 hours a day, praying they don't get laid off so they can keep their health insurance and pay their bills. (Bills their jobs are barely paying, by the way.)

I've encountered tired and stressed out single mothers who are doing everything to raise their kids alone and are having a difficult time keeping them on the straight and narrow.

I've worked on jobs where I was just going through the motions, doing what I had to do for a paycheck. Working for supervisors who knew little but thought they were better than the rest of us because of their title.

I remember feeling totally helpless as I watched my mother die a painful death from cancer. I was powerless and VERY angry. I never understood why she had to suffer like she did.

I've encountered senior citizens who seemed angry and bitter. Just mad at the world. Why? Why the anger and resentment?

But then it hit me. Too many of us are just trying to survive. We aren't living; we are surviving. There's a big difference between the two.

We grow up thinking if we do the "right" thing, we will live happily ever after. We will get that dream job if we go to college. We'll meet our dream girl (or guy), fall in love, have great kids, and life will be perfect.

We won't have to worry about bills, everyone will treat us nice and we'll never get sick.

But then we quickly realize life isn't really that way. It doesn't always go the way we expect it to.

Instead of getting that "dream job," we get a job because thanks to a poor job market, we had to take what we could find. If that isn't bad enough, we also get student loans to pay for a degree we aren't fully utilizing.

Our "perfect mate" likes to play mind games and insists on having the last word and nothing we do is good enough for them.

We go get a physical and discover we are overweight, have diabetes and borderline high blood pressure.

Before you know it, you're working long hours at a job you may or may not really care for, just to pay your bills and keep a roof over your head.

This may not be happening to you, but someone close to you may be experiencing these things. The raw realities of life are slowly setting in.

Then there are those who grew up thinking they NEVER had a chance. They live in a bad neighborhood where they are surrounded by violence, a lack of jobs, and a lack of opportunity. They were bullied and picked on for as long as they could remember. They never had a support system or anyone encouraging them to be the best they can be.

Again, this may not be you, but you may know someone in this situation.

In each of the cases above, a person can have emotions ranging from anger, sadness, depression, anxiety, low self-esteem, rage, and regret. Are these feelings justified? In my opinion, yes. Yes to an extent.

Let's just say a person is feeling any of these emotions. These feelings are gnawing at them and disrupting their day, or they have been holding onto them for years. People who are angry or depressed aren't the best of company, so these feelings might be affecting those around them.

These feelings are normal, but at the same time, the REASONS you are feeling them is many times out of your control. Yes, I watched my mother die, but as I said before, I was helpless and couldn't do anything. I held onto my anger at the world for YEARS. I was angry "just because," but what did that do for me? How did that help ME in the long run?

It didn't. It hurt me, actually. It hurt me in the fact that I moved away and lost touch with my family for years because I wasn't ready to communicate with them. They didn't know why I stopped communicating with them; they assumed that I wanted nothing to do with them.

And years later, I was finally able to go back to Chicago and I told them WHY I disappeared for years. They understood, but thought I left because I wanted nothing to do with them, which was not the case.

I lost years of family interaction because I let my anger get the best of me. Thankfully, I have reconnected with my family and we communicate often. Yes, the death of my mother hurt me, but it also hurt my interactions with my other family members for years.

How many others have let their emotions get the best of them and it affected relationships that had NOTHING to do with the reason they were upset?

How many people have gotten SICK because of letting things outside of their control affect them?

Many of the emotions we feel are the result of an outside source.

We're angry or sad because something bad happened to us. On the flipside, we're happy because something happened (or didn't happen). Or we won't be happy UNTIL something happens to us.

I give these examples to say this is NOT the way to live! For many of us, our emotions are dictated by things out of our control. Our emotions are like leaves blowing in the wind: Wherever the wind blows, that's where they'll go.

So based on my past experiences and what I've seen, I have grudgingly come to accept the fact that life really isn't fair. Things will happen to us that we don't like. Someone will say or do something we don't agree with. Our best laid plans will shatter into a million pieces. Everything we hold dear can be snatched from us.

Analyzing "why" these things happen won't help. It's done. We MUST accept what has happened, deal with it, and adjust accordingly. A person MUST have a certain mindset to survive in this world.

There are so many things out there that can break your spirit and beat you down if you let it.

IF YOU LET IT.

That's the key. If you let it! Or you can use those negative experiences as the foundation for your toughness. A springboard to help you reach your full potential. As I said before, this book was written out of anger and frustration. Matter of fact, much of this book was written in my car on my lunch break. Instead of spending my time talking about how I was unhappy and unsatisfied with my situation, I decided to do something that would help me get OUT of this situation.

I refused to accept the fact that this was my life. I was determined to take control of my life and start doing something I wanted to do. So I channeled those feelings into the words you're reading right now.

This mindset and mental toughness really started to form after the death of my mother. Do you really think you can hurt me after I watched my mother die? No, it's not possible. I am an only child who grew up without a father. I have survived that ordeal, and anything after that is NOTHING.

That's how I truly feel, and others can use the negative experiences in their lives in the same way. Either use them to make you stronger or let them keep you down.

Of course I would rather NOT have gone through that, but I did, and I can't turn back the clock. So I will use that experience in the way that helps me the most. When times are tough and I get down, I will think about those days in the hospital. I will remind myself how I made it through that, and I WILL make it through this.

I just have to keep going. WE have to keep going.

This thought process is what kept me focused on writing this book. Between working full-time, training clients, preparing for my own triathlons, and a 2-year-old at home, my time was stretched thin. But I was determined to make time for this. So, in addition to writing on my lunch breaks, I'd lay in bed at 2 am on Saturday nights, writing.

If it's really important to you, you'll make the time. You'll find a way.

We have to find some JOY while here on this earth. Joy and a sense of purpose. There MUST be something that you have to look forward to when you wake up in the morning. Life is much more than going to work, coming home, watching TV, going to bed, then waking up to repeat the cycle. We can't let our trials and tribulations stop us from being happy and living our lives to the fullest. Things WILL happen that are out of our control, but what we CAN control is how we deal with those situations. Yes, we will get knocked down, but we MUST get back up!

No one can tell you what that sense of purpose is, but if you look deep within yourself, you will find yours. For years, triathlons gave me a sense of purpose. When I became a personal trainer, helping my clients reach their fitness goals became a purpose.

Then came the birth of my son. Raising him has been added to my "Purpose List." Now, my latest purpose added to my List is the writing of this book. What will it be in the future? Time will tell, but I'll have something for sure!

If you don't have a purpose, find one!

If you already have a purpose or had a purpose and it's been changed, don't fret. I thought my original purpose was to be a financial advisor. Not just *a* financial advisor, but one of the most knowledgeable, sought after advisors out there! But that wasn't meant to be.

Life has a funny way of taking unexpected twists and turns. You expect life to go in one direction, but it veers off course in an instant. Sometimes the change is good, other times it's not. But in the midst of confusion and uncertainty, this is where our ability to change and adapt to the circumstances comes into play.

The financial industry is much different from when I became an advisor. Yes, I was upset, but spending all my time analyzing why it changed would do me no good. I had no choice but to adapt. I had to switch gears.

Animals are masters at adapting. In order to survive they adapt. The climate or habitat may change and they have no choice. Those who don't adapt become extinct. Animals don't sit around and analyze why they must change, they simply do what they have to do, or they don't make it. It's the same with us. We all know someone who is "extinct." They are living in the past, resistant to change, and stuck in their ways. They would rather reminisce about "the good old days," or hold grudges and have resentment towards those that wronged them in the past.

This book lets you know that you CAN change. You CAN adapt, and the success and happiness you deserve is possible by being physically, mentally, and spiritually fit. Even if no one else believes in you or understands what you're doing or going through, that's okay, because this your journey, no anyone else's.

Take control of your life! Strive to be the best you can be! Take care of your body so you can age gracefully and enjoy the fruits of your hard work! Understand that life can be tough, but you're tougher. Remind yourself that you are mentally strong and no matter what life throws at you, you can handle it!

And lastly, find your inner peace. Treat people with the dignity and respect you expect to receive in return. Don't degrade yourself or put others down so you can become successful. That's not what we're about! Be the inspiration and support system for those in need. Don't lose sleep wondering if you're hurting others will come back to haunt you!

This is your time, and the time is now! All it takes to get started is the mere thought and acknowledgment that you're ready to take the first step and that no one or nothing will stop you! You have all the tools deep inside you. It's time to be the best you can be!

Thank you for reading! Till next time, peace!

Jeff White

ABOUT THE AUTHOR

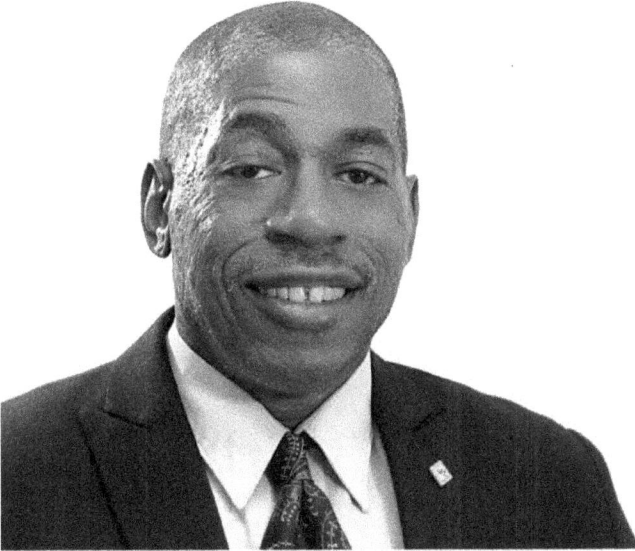

Jeffrey White is a former financial advisor turned author, personal trainer, motivational speaker and wellness coach. Jeff has been involved in fitness for more than 25 years, working as a lifeguard and completing many triathlons along the way. Jeff is from Chicago and obtained a bachelor's degree in Business Administration from Illinois State University. He believes a strong mind and body go hand in hand, and both are needed for optimum performance in all of life's endeavors. Jeffrey lives in Florida with his wife Monica and son Little Jeffrey.

www.ingramcontent.com/pod-product-compliance
Lightning Source LLC
Chambersburg PA
CBHW071347280326
41927CB00039B/2184